W9-CIH-101

Low-FODMAP and Vegan

WHAT TO EAT WHEN YOU CAN'T EAT ANYTHING

Jo Stepaniak, MSEd

Book Publishing Company
SUMMERTOWN, TENNESSEE

Library of Congress Cataloging-in-Publication Data

Names: Stepaniak, Jo, author.

Title: Low-FODMAP and vegan : what to eat when you can't eat anything / Jo
    Stepaniak, MSEd.

Other titles: Low-Fermentable Oligosaccharides, Disaccharides,
    Monosaccharides and Polyols and vegan

Description: Summertown, Tennessee : Book Publishing Company, [2016] |
    Includes index.

Identifiers: LCCN 2016005668 (print) | LCCN 2016009816 (ebook) | ISBN
    9781570673375 (pbk.) | ISBN 9781570678592 (e-book)

Subjects: LCSH: Malabsorption syndromes—Diet therapy—Recipes. | Irritable
    colon—Diet therapy—Recipes. | Veganism.

Classification: LCC RC862.M3 S74 2016 (print) | LCC RC862.M3 (ebook) | DDC
    641.5/631—dc23

LC record available at http://lccn.loc.gov/2016005668

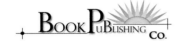

The Forest Stewardship Council® is an international nongovernmental organization that promotes environmentally appropriate, socially beneficial, and economically viable management of the world's forests. To learn more, visit www.fsc.org

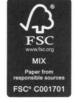

Front cover: Bliss Bowls, page 104
Back cover: Cream of Carrot and Parsnip Soup, page 122;
          Eggplant and Spinach Bolognese with Pasta, page 98

Photography and food styling: Alan Roettinger
Cover and interior design: John Wincek
Stock photography: 123 RF

Printed in China

Book Publishing Company
PO Box 99
Summertown, TN 38483
888-260-8458
bookpubco.com

ISBN: 978-1-57067-337-5

Disclaimer: The information in this book is presented for educational purposes only. It isn't intended to be a substitute for the medical advice of a physician, dietitian, or other health care professional.

CONTENTS

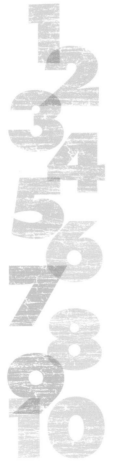

ACKNOWLEDGMENTS

My deepest gratitude to Book Publishing Company for being innovators in ethical publishing, and especially to Bob and Cynthia Holzapfel for recognizing the need for a book that addresses functional digestive disorders and vegan diets. Enormous thanks to chef Beverly Lynn Bennett for tirelessly testing a number of recipes in this book and contributing a few of her own specifically for it. Her suggestions, culinary expertise, and boundless generosity have been invaluable. I greatly appreciate the nutritional analyses done by cookbook author and recipe developer Laurie Sadowski, as well as her extremely helpful advice and constructive feedback. Many thanks to chef, cookbook author, and photographer Alan Roettinger for meticulously preparing, styling, and shooting the photos for this book, and to photographer Laura Look for her astute direction and oversight. Much gratitude to John Wincek for his infinite creativity and spectacular job with the cover and interior design.

I'm indebted to Sue Shepherd, PhD, Peter Gibson, MD, and all the amazing researchers and dieticians affiliated with the low-FODMAP diet project and app at Monash University in Australia. Thank you to dietitians Kate Scarlata, RD/RDN, and Patsy Catsos, MS, RDN, LD, who have pioneered peer education in the United States about the low-FODMAP diet and also provide clinical support to people with IBS and other digestive issues. A deep bow of appreciation to Mark Pimentel, MD, director of the Gastrointestinal Motility Program and Laboratory at Cedars-Sinai Medical Center, for his ongoing commitment to find the causes of IBS and develop effective treatments. And, of course, I'm ever grateful to the members of the vegan community and their selfless efforts to make our planet a more loving and compassionate home for all life. Finally, I extend my love and gratitude to my husband, Michael, who has not only patiently endured my digestive challenges but has also remained my champion, best friend, and intrepid taste tester.

INTRODUCTION

Nearly everyone who adopts a vegan diet, regardless of their reasons, rightfully expects to see improvements in their health. After all, eating more plant-based foods, especially whole, minimally processed foods, has been shown in study after study to benefit health in a vast number of ways. Scout the web, go to a vegan festival, attend an animal rights conference, take a vegan nutrition course, read a vegan blog or book, or listen to a vegan podcast, and you'll discover countless people who claim to have cured every ailment under the sun just by following a vegan diet.

But what if you don't feel good when you become vegan? What if your health problems take a nosedive rather than resolve? Who can you turn to if you feel worse rather than better?

Because of the well-deserved positive press that plant foods have received, it's become almost heretical to disclose that you don't feel well on a vegan diet. And if you do speak up, your vegan friends and countless others on social media will no doubt be delighted to tell you exactly what you're doing wrong and how to fix it: adopt a raw diet; go oil-free; fast; juice more; eat fewer starches; eat *more* starches; eliminate grains; ditch gluten; get more fiber; avoid sugar; go low-carb; abstain from nuts; drink green smoothies. Consequently, it's no surprise that most vegans who don't feel well are unwilling to talk about it, and it's also no surprise that many of us privately harbor an enormous amount of guilt, shame, and embarrassment about our situation. We too wonder what we're doing wrong. Why aren't we among the majority of vegans who are thriving and feeling fabulous? What's the matter with us?

I became a vegetarian when I was a child, long before it was fashionable or commonplace. And I became a vegan many decades ago, also long before it trended. I loved vegetables when I was little (yes, I was the nerdy kid who would rather eat spinach than dessert) and any food deemed healthy. And yet I never seemed to feel very good. I suffered from terrible stomachaches, headaches, and bowel issues, and rather than feel better when I became vegan, I actually felt worse.

As an adult, I tried every approach under the sun to make the pain and gut problems go away: probiotics, prebiotics, a raw diet, a high-fiber diet, juicing, nutritional supplements, fiber supplements, fasting, going gluten-free, going oil-free, going fat-free, going sugar-free, going yeast-free, going nutritarian, eating fermented foods, following food combining, doing cleanses, trying elimination diets, you name it. I tried each of these methods not just briefly on a whim but for years (as I mentioned, I've been vegan for many decades). But absolutely nothing worked.

In addition, I shuttled from doctor to doctor, trying to get a handle on what was wrong with me. I exercised. I ate well. I didn't smoke. I didn't drink alcohol or take drugs. I meditated. I had meaningful work. I should have been feeling great, right? After rounds and rounds of tests, each doctor declared that I was fit and healthy and that I "only" had irritable bowel syndrome. Then they ushered me out of their offices, dismissing me with a flick of the wrist and a subtle smirk that implied "I have patients with serious health issues. Stop bothering me."

When you're vegan and have unrelenting IBS, it's a pretty lonely and exasperating experience. I was tired of my vegan peers telling me what I should do (been there, done that) and doctors brushing me off as though IBS wasn't a "real" problem or was all in my head. And, let's face it, discussing digestive troubles isn't pretty, pleasant, or socially acceptable, so getting support and understanding, especially from people who don't have a clue what you're going through or know what it's like to live with chronic pain and discomfort, fear about embarrassing yourself, and anxiety over where to find the nearest bathroom is particularly challenging.

But after many years of suffering and many years of research, I finally hit upon something that has helped. And because of that, I'm stepping out of the water closet to share my discoveries and reveal (rather reluctantly) that I'm vegan and I have IBS. No longer should those of us with functional digestive disorders suffer in silence or be ashamed of being vegan and not feeling well.

I offer this book to you unapologetically, my friend: the vegan with IBS. I also offer it to any vegan with other functional digestive disorders and related gastrointestinal conditions, including inflammatory bowel disease (Crohn's disease and ulcerative colitis), celiac disease, and those with "sensitive stomachs." If you've ever had days (or weeks, or months, or years) when you've felt you're essentially allergic to food and can't eat anything at all, this book is for you.

Although there currently is no cure for IBS, we can learn how to pinpoint triggers and manage our symptoms through a revolutionary, scientifically proven method. I invite you to turn the page and join me on this exciting journey.

Jo Stepaniak
ibsvegan.com

Understanding IBS

Irritable bowel syndrome (IBS) is a chronic, common disorder that affects about 10 percent of the world's population and 10 to 15 percent of the general population in the United States, including women and men of all ages. According to the Canadian Digestive Health Foundation, IBS affects 18 percent of the population in Canada, one of the highest rates in the world. The Gastrointestinal Society of Canada and the Canadian Society of Intestinal Research state that the lifetime risk for a Canadian to develop IBS is 30 percent. Despite these startling numbers, it's estimated that fewer than 15 percent of people worldwide who are affected by IBS seek medical attention.

IBS mainly involves the large intestine (colon) and is characterized by cramping, recurrent abdominal pain, altered bowel habits, bloating, abdominal distention, excessive gas and flatulence, variations in stool characteristics, audible abdominal noises or rumbling (the noises are called "borborygmi"), fecal urgency, unsatisfied defecation (a sensation of incomplete emptying), mucus in the stools, rectal pain, nausea, and fatigue. For most people, IBS is a persistent, unrelenting condition, although there will likely be times when the signs and symptoms are worse and times when they improve or even disappear completely.

Upper GI symptoms, such as belching, dysphagia (difficulty swallowing), dyspepsia (indigestion), heartburn, noncardiac chest pain, and increased gas production are also common in people with IBS. Extraintestinal (non-gastrointestinal) symptoms that are frequently reported include rheumatologic symptoms (inflammation or pain in muscles, joints, or fibrous tissue), headaches (including migraines), increased urinary frequency and urgency, sexual dysfunction, and sleep-related disturbances. There also appears to be a strong connection between IBS and fibromyalgia (chronic muscle aches and pain). In his paper titled "The Association of Irritable

Bowel Syndrome and Fibromyalgia," Lin Chang, MD, associate professor of medicine, co-director of the UCLA/CURE Neuroenteric Disease Program, and director of the UCLA Motility Unit, reported that up to 60 percent of people diagnosed with fibromyalgia have symptoms of IBS and up to 70 percent of people diagnosed with IBS have symptoms of fibromyalgia. The similar clinical characteristics and significant overlap of symptoms between these two syndromes suggest that they may have a common etiology. Most notable, however, is that the primary clinical pattern of IBS—the chronic abdominal pain and altered bowel habits—hasn't been explained by any identifiable structural or biochemical abnormalities, as it has with inflammatory bowel diseases, such as Crohn's disease and ulcerative colitis. While some research shows that the colons of IBS sufferers have similar physical characteristics, for the most part IBS has been defined by its lack of verifiable criteria. Nevertheless, having a diagnosis of IBS does not mean the symptoms are any less real than for patients with organic or structural diagnoses. In fact, research has shown that the severity of the symptoms and degree of disability for many IBS patients are even greater than for patients with ulcers, esophageal reflux, or milder forms of inflammatory bowel disease.

Because the pathophysiology of IBS has not been entirely clear, it has made diagnosis and treatment challenging. It's also the main reason that IBS has long been dismissed as a psychosomatic condition. Traditionally, doctors have diagnosed IBS by exclusion, which means that rather than making a positive diagnosis of IBS, they've relied on ruling out the presence of other conditions and illnesses, such as colorectal disease, colon cancer, celiac disease, and inflammatory bowel disease (IBD). Since IBS is a disorder of abnormal gut functioning, no abnormalities should show up on the various conventional diagnostic tests that are used, so negative test results only help to reinforce this diagnosis. In addition to investigative tests, the diagnostic process typically includes identification of symptoms suggestive of IBS, known as the ABC of IBS:

A Abdominal pain or cramping
B Bloating or a feeling of fullness
C Changes in bowel habits:
   - more than three bowel movements per day or fewer than three bowel movements per week
   - change in stool form or appearance (e.g., lumpy/hard stool, pellets, pencil-like stool, unformed stool, loose and/or watery stool)
   - change in stool passage (e.g., straining, urgency, or a feeling of incomplete emptying)

The official medical definition of IBS is part of what is known as the Rome IV Diagnostic Criteria for Functional Gastrointestinal Disorders. This criteria system was developed to classify functional gastrointestinal disorders based on clinical symptoms. The Rome IV diagnostic criteria for irritable bowel syndrome states the following:

> Symptoms of recurrent abdominal pain and a marked change in bowel habits for at least six months, with recurrent abdominal pain at least three days a month during the last three months associated with two or more of the following:
>
> - Pain is relieved by a bowel movement
> - Onset is associated with a change in frequency of stool
> - Onset is associated with a change in form (appearance) of stool

Despite the prevalence of the syndrome, the exact cause of IBS still isn't known. The current clinical understanding is that it is a disorder primarily resulting from the confluence and interaction of several elements: visceral hypersensitivity (increased sensitivity to pain in the intestines), genetics, infection (such as food poisoning), inflammation, and gut motility. Other possible influences include dietary factors, gastrointestinal dysmotility (impaired muscles in the GI tract), gastrointestinal dysfunction (increased or decreased contractions of the digestive organs), imbalanced gut flora (bacterial overgrowth in the large intestine), small intestinal bacterial overgrowth (SIBO), hormones, and environmental and psychological elements.

However, some exciting and encouraging medical breakthroughs in research and testing for IBS have recently occurred: Scientists have identified an organic biomarker for the diagnosis of one type of IBS. The tests, created by Mark Pimentel, MD, director of the GI Motility Program and Laboratory at Cedars-Sinai Medical Center, confirm when a patient has developed IBS because of food poisoning, which is one of the major causes of the disorder. (Ten percent, and possibly more, of IBS cases seem to occur after an acute bout of food poisoning.) The blood tests identified the two antibodies associated with diarrhea-predominant IBS (IBS-D)—anti-Cdtb and anti-vinculin—with greater than 90 percent certainty. Toxins produced by foodborne bacteria, such as *Salmonella* or *Shigella,* can severely harm the digestive tract by damaging nerves critical to healthy gut function. The new blood tests, marketed under the name IBSchek and produced by Commonwealth Laboratories Inc. in Salem, Massachusetts, identify the presence and amount of specific antibodies reacting to the toxins.

The initial test is specific to IBS-D, but a similar test for constipation-predominant IBS is on the horizon. Being able to identify the organic biomarkers and mechanisms of IBS means that researchers will be able to develop better and more effective treatment options targeted to each specific type of IBS. It also means that early diagnosis will help shorten the time of investigation, help patients avoid invasive testing and the need to go from doctor to doctor, and accelerate access to treatment.

THE POOP ON IBS

- It's estimated that worldwide IBS affects from 1 in 10 to nearly 1 in 4 people (9 percent to 23 percent of the world's population).

- IBS affects 10 to 15 percent of the population in the United States, or between 25 and 45 million people.

- IBS affects about 18 percent of the population in Canada, or about 5 million people, one of the highest rates in the world.

- Women are at greater risk than men of developing IBS; it occurs in almost twice as many women as men.

- IBS affects people of all ages, even children. Although most people with IBS are under the age of fifty, many older adults suffer from IBS as well.

- IBS is the second most-common cause of work and school absenteeism. (The first is the common cold.)

- A gastrointestinal infection can instigate or worsen IBS. This is called post-infectious IBS.

- The exact cause of IBS is not known. Symptoms may result from a disturbance in the way the gut, brain, and nervous system interact. This can cause changes in normal bowel movements and visceral sensations.

- Stress does not cause IBS. However, because of the close connection between the brain and gut, stress can trigger or worsen symptoms.

- The effects of IBS can range from mild inconvenience to severe debilitation. Long-term symptoms can disrupt and negatively impact a person's emotional, social, educational, and professional well-being.

- IBS is unpredictable. Symptoms typically vary and are often contradictory. For example, diarrhea can alternate with constipation.

- Despite the prevalence of IBS, few people seek medical treatment, and a diagnosis typically isn't made until several years after the onset of symptoms.

- IBS does not damage the intestines or lead to cancer. It is not related to inflammatory bowel disease (IBD), such as Crohn's disease and ulcerative colitis.

In addition, having such a test brings relief and validation to the millions of IBS sufferers who have lived in doubt of and shame about their ailment.

If the result of the blood test is positive, your doctor will know the reason you have IBS and can use a targeted treatment approach. However, a negative or inconclusive result may not necessarily mean that you don't have IBS. It may simply be an indication that your doctor needs to conduct further testing to ascertain the cause of your symptoms and determine whether there is an alternative mechanism responsible for them.

Also, new research by the American Academy of Neurology in 2016 revealed that in patients with IBS-C, serotonin secretion in plasma is decreased and that there is a defect in serotonin signaling. Additionally, the research found that patients with IBS, migraines, or tension headaches all had at least one gene that was different from those in the healthy controls, suggesting that these three conditions may share a genetic link. Because IBS and headaches are so common, and because the causes of these conditions are unknown, finding a connection that could illuminate their shared genetics is encouraging.

Although IBS can be debilitating and disruptive and can negatively affect quality of life, there is no evidence that it leads to more serious or life-threatening conditions, causes structural damage to the gastrointestinal tract, or shortens a person's life span. However, because the symptoms of IBS frequently mimic those of other ailments, it's vital to have a confirmed diagnosis from a physician rather than attempt to self-diagnose. Your doctor will try to identify red-flag symptoms that might indicate conditions other than IBS by asking targeted questions:

- Did the onset of symptoms occur after age fifty?
- Is there blood in your stool?
- Do you have a fever?
- Have you had unintentional weight loss of more than ten pounds?
- Do your symptoms wake you up at night?
- Do you have a family history of colorectal cancer?

If no other disease or injury can be found as a source of the gastrointestinal symptoms, or if you receive a positive blood test result, IBS may be diagnosed, falling into one of four categories:

- IBS with diarrhea (IBS-D): Diarrhea (loose stools) is the most frequent symptom.
- IBS with constipation (IBS-C): Constipation or hard stools is the most frequent symptom.
- IBS mixed or IBS alternating (IBS-M or IBS-A): Both constipation and diarrhea are experienced alternately.
- IBS unspecified (IBS-U): Symptoms follow an irregular pattern.

Previously, IBS was defined by the absence of structural disease. However, the updated Rome IV criteria revised that definition and now includes it under disorders of GI functioning, specifically disorders of gut-brain interaction. These disorders are classified by GI symptoms related to any combination of the following:

- Motility disturbance
- Visceral hypersensitivity
- Altered mucosal and immune function
- Altered gut microbiota
- Altered central nervous system (CNS) processing

Once a firm diagnosis of IBS is made, your doctor can assist you with developing a treatment plan that will help you manage your symptoms, pinpoint triggers, and avoid possible complications from problems such as chronic diarrhea. You might also get a referral to a dietitian familiar with vegan and low-FODMAP diets or an endorsement to try a low-FODMAP diet as outlined in this book.

Treating IBS

It's important for people diagnosed with IBS to proactively take control of their health and general well-being. Because there currently is no cure for IBS, the key to successful treatment is symptom management. Fortunately, there are a number of helpful approaches you can pursue right now to assist in that regard.

Lifestyle Changes

The easiest and most crucial first step in getting a handle on your IBS is to determine which important lifestyle changes you need to make.

Exercise. Regular exercise has been shown to ease IBS symptoms. While it's not necessary to run a marathon, it may be beneficial to stretch, take brisk walks, and do simple exercises at home or at the gym. Aim for at least thirty minutes of exercise every day. Build exercise into your daily routine by taking the stairs whenever possible, going for a walk at lunchtime, or walking or biking instead of driving or taking public transportation. When feasible, park a distance from your destination and walk the remainder of the journey.

Manage stress. Although stress and other emotional factors are not the cause of IBS, they may trigger or worsen symptoms in some people. Meditation, yoga, and other forms of stress relief may help keep stress levels in check and emotions on an even keel.

Get enough sleep. Sleep-related disturbances are often an IBS symptom, but the irony is that exhaustion can exacerbate symptoms further. Make it a goal to get sufficient sleep each night, and stick to a routine of waking up and going to bed at the same time every day.

Keep a food and symptom diary. It's often helpful to keep a thorough, detailed food and symptom diary for two to four weeks to monitor your eating habits, lifestyle, and activities. Doing so will help you identify triggers (see page 12) and the severity of the symptoms they produce and determine whether certain treatments (such as exercise, medications, stress management, supplements, or diet modifications) are helping.

Dietary Habits

When you have IBS, *how* you eat is as important as *what* you eat. While the chapters that follow will cover in detail what to eat and what to avoid and why, the tips below will help you navigate some additional dietary terrain:

Schedule regular meals. Have your meals at the same times every day, and eat at a leisurely, unhurried pace. Avoid using mealtimes for difficult discussions or stress-filled conversations.

Don't skip meals. Avoid missing meals or leaving long gaps between eating. Hunger can aggravate a sensitive gut, entice you to eat rapidly, tempt you to chow down on whatever is handy (even if it's a trigger food), and cause you to overeat. Plan your breakfast in advance so you have something to look forward to in the morning. A wholesome breakfast can increase alertness and decrease the urge to snack during the day. Include nutrient-dense and/or fiber-rich foods at breakfast, as these can make you feel satiated longer.

Eat smaller meals. Large meals and overeating are known IBS triggers. In addition, eating small meals means you will consume fewer trigger foods at a pop. Aim for smaller but more frequent meals. If you find it hard to regulate portions, buy smaller plates, bowls, and glasses. This can help you to easily reduce portion sizes and decrease caloric intake.

Plan ahead. Assemble your lunch the night before or get up a little earlier in the morning to put it together. Also prepare small snacks and portion them in ziplock bags. This way, when you're hungry during the day, you'll have something healthy and safe to eat, and you can avoid the need to just grab whatever is handy, which might cause a flare-up.

Hydrate. Drink at least eight cups of fluids per day. Water and clear liquids, such as unsweetened, caffeine-free herbal tea (especially ginger or peppermint tea, both of which can assist with calming and soothing a temperamental digestive system), will help keep the stool soft, making it easier for it to move through the intestinal tract. Note that certain herbal products and teas can interact with some medications (for example, peppermint can interfere with acid-reducing drugs or aggravate reflux disease), so talk with your health care provider before using herbal teas if you're taking any medications or have been diagnosed with GERD or hiatal hernia.

Fiber

It has long been believed and promoted that all anyone with IBS needs to do is "eat more fiber." Unfortunately, many physicians and dietitians are still advising this approach to their patients despite there being little evidence that more fiber in the diet benefits IBS symptoms or that too little fiber is a cause of IBS. And misguided friends and family will no doubt continue to offer up similar advice.

Generally speaking, vegans who eat a diet of mostly whole, minimally processed foods are already getting plenty of fiber. Foods rich in insoluble fiber include bran from whole-grain cereals and breads, cruciferous vegetables, and the skin of root vegetables (such as potatoes) and many kinds of fruit. Insoluble fiber can cause more harm than good in people with a hypersensitive gut because this type of fiber tends to cause fermentation, which can lead to bloating and gas, resulting in abdominal cramping and pain in people with IBS.

Soluble fiber is another type of fiber found in a broad range of foods, such as apples, legumes (beans, peas, and lentils), and oats. Soluble fiber attracts water and forms a gel that sweeps along the gut and helps to move the bowels. For people with IBS-C (constipation-predominant IBS), soluble fiber can help ease constipation. However, in people with IBS-D (diarrhea-predominant IBS), IBS-M or IBS-A (IBS with alternating constipation and diarrhea), and IBS-U (unsubtyped IBS), this type of fiber can exacerbate symptoms. In addition, foods that contain soluble fiber often are rich in fermentable carbohydrates known as FODMAPs (see page 15) that can wreak havoc on a sensitive gut.

Consequently, the knee-jerk admonition to just "eat more fiber" isn't as simple, safe, or smart for people with IBS as it may sound. In fact, if you are constipated and are consuming a large amount of fiber in your diet, *decreasing* the amount of fiber you ingest might actually help ease some of your IBS symptoms.

When you don't feel well or are having a flare-up, drinking more clear liquids, blending foods (which helps break down their fiber), and eating soft, well-cooked, low-fiber foods can soothe an irritable gut. Although most nutrition experts advise getting nutrients, including fiber, from food rather than supplements, IBS sufferers may find that a diet high in fiber causes more cramping, gas, pain, and other symptoms than a lower-fiber diet with supplemental low-FODMAP fiber. If you find that a low-fiber diet helps relieve your symptoms, you can try adding nonfermentable fiber supplements, such as psyllium husks or powder (see Resources, page 133), to your daily regimen, starting with a very small dose and increasing the amount gradually over time. Supplements made of cellulose (methylcellulose) are also worth trying, since that type of fiber is not fermentable. Avoid fiber supplements made with inulin (also known as chicory root; see page 13) or processed foods with fiber added to them, as these tend to worsen symptoms.

Other Approaches

Probiotics

Probiotics are nutritional supplements and fermented or cultured foods (such as yogurt) that contain friendly bacteria. They are purported to improve the intestinal flora by balancing the ratio of "good" to "bad" bacteria, which may benefit digestion and have a positive effect on IBS symptoms. At present, the types of bacterial strains used in probiotic products vary greatly. Further research is needed to clarify the role and value of probiotics and, if proven useful, determine which strains are the most helpful.

Probiotics need to be taken daily, as they don't remain in the gut for long. A 2015 study out of Moscow showed statistically significant improvement in symptoms for both IBS-D and IBS-C using a combination of *Bifidobacterium bifidum, Bifidobacterium longum, Bifidobacterium infantis,* and *Lactobacillus rhamnosus.* With additional positive research, specific probiotic combinations like this could become valuable assets in IBS treatment. Other than the cost, probiotics in recommended dosages shouldn't do any harm. If you want to give probiotics a try, do so for four to six weeks. If you don't see any improvement in your IBS symptoms, discontinue them.

To ensure that the probiotic supplement you purchase actually contains live bacteria, pour ½ cup of soymilk into a small container. Open three or four probiotic capsules (look for probiotics in veggie caps) and sprinkle the contents over the soymilk. Stir well and let rest at room temperature for 8 to 10 hours. If the soymilk clumps, curdles, or thickens, the bacteria in the probiotic are alive and kicking. If the soymilk remains unchanged, the bacteria is inactive and shouldn't be used.

Prebiotics

Prebiotics are nondigestible carbohydrates that act as food for probiotics and stimulate the growth of beneficial gut microbiota. Because foods that contain these nondigestible carbohydrates, known as FODMAPs (see page 15), are prebiotics, they support this good bacteria and help to maintain a healthy balance in the gut. A reduction of these foods generally improves IBS symptoms because they ferment and produce gas. However, recent studies conducted at King's College in London and at Monash University in Australia have shown that individuals who stay on a diet that's very low in FODMAPs for long stretches develop changes in their gut microbiota that result in lower levels of beneficial bacteria. The study of the gut microbiome is a relatively new area of research, and scientists don't yet fully understand the implications of the long-term changes a low-FODMAP diet can cause to the balance of friendly bacteria. For that reason, staying on a very restricted, very low-FODMAP diet for an extended period or lifetime isn't advisable (see Reintroducing FODMAPs, page 38). Nevertheless, there is no evidence to date that prebiotic supplements help with IBS and instead are more likely to instigate and exacerbate the symptoms of functional digestive disorders.

Nutritional Supplements

While some IBS sufferers claim relief from certain nutritional supplements, such as magnesium, omega-3 fatty acids, zinc, and vitamins B, C, and D, there is no peer-reviewed evidence to date for the benefit of these therapies. Nevertheless, intestinal disorders can cause mineral imbalances, and limited diets can cause vitamin and mineral deficiencies, so you might find some benefit from supplementation.

There is substantial anecdotal evidence that magnesium supplementation, particularly magnesium citrate (see Resources, page 133), can benefit IBS-C. If you want to try it, start with a low dose of 50 to 250 milligrams of magnesium citrate per day with food and gradually increase the dose as needed until good bowel function resumes. If you find that magnesium citrate is beneficial, it may take a little time and experimentation to find the right maintenance dose. A common standard dose is 400 milligrams per day, or 200 milligrams twice a day, but you might require more or less than that. There are many other types of magnesium, but they won't all have the same effects and some may require a different dosage. If magnesium supplementation causes loose stools or diarrhea, decrease the dose or stop taking it altogether.

Magnesium glycinate typically doesn't have the same effect on the bowels as magnesium citrate, but it may help more with muscle relaxation and aid sleep, especially when taken at bedtime. Magnesium malate, a compound of magnesium and malic acid, is purported to help relieve pain, improve bowel function, increase energy, and benefit sleep. (See Resources, page 133.)

Again, the amount of magnesium you may need to help relieve your symptoms might be higher or lower than what is commonly recommended, and different types of magnesium may work better for you than others. Be sure to discuss your plans with your doctor before starting on nutritional supplements, because some supplements can interact negatively with other medications or cause toxicity or undesirable side effects, especially in inappropriate dosages.

Psychological Therapies

Many people with IBS explore psychological approaches, such as hypnotherapy, cognitive behavioral therapy, and mindfulness-based stress reduction, to deal with stress related to their condition and anxiety that could be contributing to their symptoms. There is evidence that these techniques may be beneficial, even for people with IBS who aren't experiencing overt stress or anxiety, and because these modalities aren't invasive or harmful, you might find it valuable to look into them.

Gluten-Free Diets

Although a gluten-free diet is often recommended as a way to treat IBS, there's currently no scientific evidence to support this. When IBS improves on a gluten-free diet, it's likely due to the elimination of fructans (see page 17), which are fermentable carbohydrates found in foods that naturally contain gluten and have been shown to exacerbate IBS symptoms. Unless a person has celiac disease, gluten intolerance, or wheat allergy, there is no need for people with IBS to specifically avoid gluten. (See page 27 for further information.)

Medications

Currently there are no approved pharmaceuticals that have been shown to relieve all IBS symptoms in all people. Rather, most drugs target just one specific problem or one specific type of IBS (either IBS-D or IBS-C), and they often come with side effects. With the advent of new testing modalities, however, this may change in the near future. In the meantime, certain medications can play a valuable role in treating or alleviating particularly troublesome IBS symptoms, including abdominal cramps and pain, diarrhea, constipation, sleep disturbances, anxiety and stress, and depression.

Common Food-Related Triggers

One of the most difficult and confounding aspects of dealing with IBS is trying to figure out which foods make symptoms worse, because specific triggers can vary somewhat from person to person. Fortunately, the low-FODMAP diet, which is discussed in the next chapter, can help enormously in this regard. In addition, there are other known food-related triggers that affect a large number of IBS sufferers:

Alcohol. Because it is an intestinal irritant, alcohol can worsen the symptoms of IBS. Limit alcoholic beverages to one standard drink per day and try to abstain from alcohol at least two days per week. When you do have a drink, have it with food rather than on an empty stomach, because food will slow down the release of alcohol from the stomach.

Artificial sweeteners. Sugar substitutes, known as artificial sweeteners, are substances used instead of sucrose (table sugar) to sweeten foods and beverages. Artificial sweeteners are made from sugar alcohols, or polyols (see page 18), such as erythritol, maltitol, sorbitol, xylitol, and numerous others, which are types of sweet carbohydrates found naturally in foods or processed from other sugars. The body cannot digest most polyols, so they travel to the large intestine where they are metabolized by the gut bacteria and can cause significant digestive distress, including gas, bloating, and diarrhea. Sugar alcohols are commonly added to "sugar-free" beverages, candies, chewing gums, and similar items. Read labels carefully and avoid products that contain these or other artificial sweeteners.

Caffeine. Caffeine naturally increases the motility of the gut, often causing painful spasms and diarrhea. If you must have caffeinated coffee or tea, limit your intake to one cup per day and avoid "energy drinks" completely.

Carbonated (fizzy) beverages. Carbonation fills the digestive tract with air, further contributing to gas and bloating and worsening IBS symptoms. Avoid all carbonated beverages, including club soda and sparkling water. While you're at it, skip the straw too, as it can force more air into the digestive tract and create additional gas.

Chewing gum. A consequence of chewing gum is swallowing excess air, which can contribute to abdominal pain and bloating. In addition, the artificial sweeteners (see page 12) used in "sugar-free" gums can cause adverse gastrointestinal symptoms, especially in people with IBS.

Fat. Fatty and fried foods are difficult to digest and can lead to gas, cramping, bloating, and diarrhea by increasing secretions to the small and large intestines. In addition to fried foods, which are fairly easy to avoid, limit consumption of nuts, nut butters, vegan mayonnaise, vegan butter (margarine), coconut (including coconut oil and coconut butter), vegetable oils, and rich desserts.

Hot chiles. Spicy foods typically contain hot chiles, which are rich in capsaicin, a naturally occurring compound. Capsaicin can irritate the mouth, stomach, and digestive tract, and for many IBS sufferers, it can also trigger symptoms. If you like spicy foods, enjoy them in moderation or turn the heat level down a notch or two, especially if hot spices aggravate your symptoms.

Inulin (chicory). Also known as chicory root, inulin is a fermentable dietary fiber that is a common IBS trigger. Read product labels carefully and avoid products that list inulin, chicory root, or chicory root fiber as an ingredient. Also avoid chicory-based coffee substitutes.

Resistant starch. Resistant starch (RS) is a type of starch that isn't fully broken down and absorbed in the stomach or small intestine and reaches the colon intact, making it "resistant" to digestion. Once RS reaches the large intestine, bacteria ferment the starch and produce gas. In many ways, resistant starch is similar to and behaves like fermentable fiber and FODMAPs (see page 15) in the digestive tract and is a common IBS trigger. Undercooked or cooked and then cooled or dried high-starch plant foods, such as potatoes (think potato salad and instant mashed potatoes), sweet potatoes, dried pastas, and rice (think rice salads and fried rice), contain more resistant starch than fully cooked hot or warm fresh foods. Additional sources of resistant starch include legumes, unripe bananas, raw potatoes, potato starch, processed foods (such as cakes, cookies, chips, and crackers), breads, cashews, and raw oats, just to name a few. If you have difficulty digesting resistant starch, try minimizing your consumption of foods with RS, cook starchy foods thoroughly, and avoid eating leftover potatoes, rice, and other cooked-then-chilled high-starch foods.

Sugar. Sugar, even the natural sugars found in fruits, can speed gut motility and aggravate IBS symptoms. Don't overdo sugar and fruits and avoid concentrated sources, including fruit juices, fruit juice concentrates, dried fruits, candies, and syrups.

FLAVOR WITHOUT FAT

Fat enhances the taste of food, infuses flavors throughout a dish, boosts satiety, and improves the absorption of fat-soluble vitamins, so many of the recipes in this book include fat in modest quantities. But fat is also a common trigger for people suffering with IBS. If fat is a trigger for you, limit the amount of fat you have at meal, use water or Good-to-Your-Gut Vegetable Stock (page 58) rather than oil for cooking and stir-frying, and keep nuts and their butters to a minimum. In addition, season your foods with low-FODMAP fat-free options, such as scallion greens, fresh and dried herbs, spices, and spice blends that are free of onion and garlic (as these are also IBS triggers). Excellent fat-free choices are All-Purpose Herb Blend (page 55), Tan-Tan Spice Mix (page 55), Sweet-n-Savory

Spice Mix (page 55), Good-to-Your-Gut Ketchup (page 57), Good-to-Your-Gut Sriracha Sauce (page 56), tamari, balsamic vinegar, and rice vinegar.

In fact, vinegars in general make ideal fat-free seasonings, but of particular note are flavored balsamics (see Resources, page 133), which can range from sweet to fruity to citrusy to spicy. Chocolate and strawberry balsamics are swoon-worthy when drizzled over almond-milk ice cream or yogurt, cantaloupe, kiwi, pineapple, or strawberries. Lemon and chile balsamics add a jolt of flavor to vegetables as well as rice and other gluten-free grains. And high-quality pomegranate, traditional dark, and white (also called "golden") balsamic vinegars make exquisite salad dressings on their own.

The Better You Eat the Worse You Feel

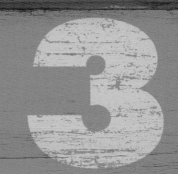

If you're vegan and have IBS, there are some valid, scientifically sound reasons why you probably feel worse the better you eat. It's definitely not all in your head.

Many plant foods acclaimed for being supernutritious, superdelicious, or simply useful in mimicking the flavors and textures of meat, cheese, and other animal products are ubiquitous in vegan dishes, but they aren't necessarily kind to IBS sufferers. It's almost impossible to find a vegan recipe, prepared item, packaged product, or frozen food that doesn't contain at least one of the ingredients at right.

And yet you probably weren't aware that these items are high up on the IBS "top triggers" list. Sadly, very few people are (including food manufacturers, chefs, restaurant owners, and vegans in general). So it's not surprising that when vegans with IBS chow down on vegan chili, nosh on nut cheese, dip into hummus, tuck into a veggie burger, bite into a burrito, nibble black-bean brownies, gobble up guacamole, chomp on cashew cheesecake, or slurp date-sweetened smoothies, their abdomens balloon like blimps and they double over in pain, bolt to the bathroom, or dash out the door to avoid an embarrassing situation.

All of these plant-based foods, as well as many others, have something in common that can bring people with IBS crumpling to their knees, begging for mercy and relief: FODMAPs. The word "FODMAP" is an acronym that stands for fermentable oligosaccharides (fructans and galacto-oligosaccharides, also known as GOS), disaccharides (lactose), monosaccharides (fructose), and polyols (polydextrose, isomalt, maltitol, mannitol, sorbitol, and xylitol). This group of naturally occurring but indigestible sugars (carbohydrates) is rapidly broken down (fermented) by bacteria in the bowel. Because these sugars aren't well absorbed in the small intestine, they pass directly through to the colon, where they then cause bowel distention by drawing in more liquid and generating gas when the bowel bacteria ferment them.

The concept of FODMAPs was conceived through research at Monash University in Melbourne, Australia. Led by Peter Gibson, director of gastroenterology at The

"top triggers"

agave nectar
apples
artichokes
avocados
beans
cashews
cauliflower
dates
garlic
mushrooms
onions
peas
pistachios
wheat

Alfred Hospital and Monash University, and Jane Muir, head of translational nutrition science at Monash University, the team became the first group in the world to measure the majority of FODMAPs in food. Today they have a comprehensive database of the FODMAP content in a wide range of foods, which has been generated out of their laboratory at the university. All the foods in their database have been rigorously tested and measured to ensure the information is accurate and based on scientific laboratory evidence rather than guesswork or anecdotal speculation. Their research is reflected in the dietary information and recipes provided in this book.

In 1999, Sue Shepherd, an Australian dietitian and researcher, developed the low-FODMAP diet, based on the database produced by the Monash University team. This revolutionary dietary therapy has been widely reviewed in international medical journals and is recommended as one of the most effective approaches for managing the symptoms of IBS. Shepherd's research demonstrated that three out of four people with IBS (about 75 percent of IBS sufferers) are helped by a low-FODMAP diet. In addition, the diet shows promise for treating the persistent symptoms of other gastrointestinal disorders and diseases, including Crohn's disease and ulcerative colitis.

While everyone has some difficulty digesting and absorbing FODMAPs, people with IBS experience cramping, pain, bloating, excessive gas, abdominal distension, altered bowel habits (including diarrhea and/or constipation), nausea, and other heightened symptoms that the general population doesn't, or doesn't nearly to the same degree. Because FODMAPs are carbohydrates, they are present only in plant foods and many dairy products; they aren't present in meat, fish, fowl, hard cheeses, or eggs, all of which are carbohydrate-free. This helps explain why some people who abandon veganism for meat-centered, low-carb diets (such as the paleo diet) claim they feel much better than they did when they were vegan. The fact is, they probably *do* feel better, particularly if they have IBS or other functional digestive problems, and there's a substantial amount of scientific evidence to back them up. Rather than condemn people who flee a vegan diet for the dark side, it would probably be more productive to try to understand their motivations. If they have functional digestive disorders, it's possible they didn't relinquish their ethics but were simply desperate to be healthy and pain-free and couldn't accomplish that on a vegan diet. It's vital to acknowledge that people with IBS have a much more difficult time thriving solely on plant foods, and their reasons are legitimate and real.

Also know that a low-FODMAP diet isn't a cure for IBS. The condition will still persist regardless of what you eat, and you'll likely continue to have symptoms to varying degrees. However, the low-FODMAP diet can be of enormous benefit because it helps IBS sufferers identify and eliminate many food-related triggers and, by doing so, better manage their symptoms.

Size Matters

Because various FODMAPs exist in all edible plants, multiple types are present in vegan foods and their repercussions are cumulative. This means that if you eat a variety of

FODMAPs in an assortment of dishes at a meal, the effects on the bowel will be compounded. That's why it's vital to take into consideration not just the amount of a single FODMAP in a single food but also the totality of all FODMAPs per serving in a prepared dish as well as in the other foods consumed with it at the meal. It's also critical to limit portion size, because large amounts of even IBS-safe foods will push the amount of FODMAPs ingested over the tolerable limit and into the danger zone.

While it's not possible to have an entirely FODMAP-free vegan diet, because virtually all plant foods contain some measure of FODMAPs, we can center our diets around foods that contain minimal amounts of FODMAPs and that aren't generally problematic (in appropriate portions) for most people with IBS. Although it's recommended to consult a registered dietitian before starting on any diet that eliminates broad groups of foods, the range of suitable plant-based foods on a low-FODMAP diet is more than sufficient to cover most nutrient needs for most vegans.

Note that the amount of a particular FODMAP in a food is what determines that food's suitability on a low-FODMAP diet. Some foods high in FODMAPs may be tolerated in very small amounts because those limited portions keep the FODMAPs in the safe zone. Bear in mind, however, that foods moderately high in FODMAPs may become intolerable in quantities larger than those recommended or when combined with other foods rich in FODMAPs that are consumed at the same meal. Portion control is important. When it comes to FODMAPs, size really does matter.

FODMAPs Deconstructed

Below is a breakdown of each group of FODMAPs and some general information about them. When you initially embark on a low-FODMAP diet, it's especially important to avoid all FODMAPs, regardless of which category they fall into. Although it's possible to have more or less sensitivity to one group of FODMAPs than another, every category has the potential to be problematic for people with IBS. This is particularly true if several foods in a group are consumed at one time or if a single food is consumed in excess. In addition, some foods contain more than one type of FODMAP, so it's not always easy to tell which FODMAP group is responsible for symptoms.

Oligosaccharides: Fructans and GOS

This category of FODMAPs is broken down into two subgroups: fructans and galacto-oligosaccharides (GOS). Fructans encompass a broad range of foods, including certain grains (wheat, rye, and barley), certain vegetables (such as garlic and onion), legumes (beans, lentils, and peas), some fruits, some nuts and seeds, and inulin (chicory root), which is added to a variety of prepared foods as a texturizer or prebiotic (see page 10). The most common galacto-oligosaccharides are raffinose and stachyose, which are present in most legumes.

Disaccharides

There is only one FODMAP in the disaccharides group: lactose. Because vegans don't consume animal-based foods, including dairy products, this category of FODMAPs is eliminated by default for vegans. However, many dairy alternatives, including soymilk and various types of nondairy milks, vegan cheeses, vegan yogurts, vegan ice creams, and a large number of other products designed to replace dairy foods may contain other high-FODMAP ingredients. Read labels carefully. Note that products made with soy protein isolate or extract (including certain brands of soymilks, soy cheeses, soy yogurts, soy creamers, and so forth), rather than whole soybeans, are low in FODMAPs and can be valuable additions to a low-FODMAP vegan diet.

Monosaccharides

There is only one FODMAP in the monosaccharides group: fructose. Often referred to as "fruit sugar," fructose is found in all fruits and fruit juice concentrates, although it's particularly high in certain fruits, such as apples, cherries, pears, and watermelon. In addition, fructose is a component of agave nectar, honey (which isn't vegan), and high-fructose corn syrup. Fructose is also found in cane sugar (although a moderate amount of cane sugar is generally well tolerated by people with IBS), grains (such as wheat), and some vegetables (such as artichokes, asparagus, and sugar snap peas).

About one in three people have what's known as fructose malabsorption, which doesn't occur with any greater frequency in people with IBS than in the general population. People with fructose malabsorption have a more difficult time absorbing excess fructose. As long as a fruit (or other fructose-containing food) also contains glucose in an equal or greater amount, even people with fructose malabsorption should be able to consume it in moderation. Whether or not you have fructose malabsorption, if you have IBS, limit fruit portions to about one medium piece (approximately the size of an orange, or ½ to 1 cup of sliced or cubed fruit, or ¾ cup of berries) at a time, and wait at least two to three hours between each serving.

Polyols

Also known as sugar alcohols, polyols are commonly given names that end in "ol," which makes them easy to recognize. These include sorbitol, mannitol, maltitol, and xylitol, as well as polydextrose and isomalt. Polyols occur naturally in some fruits (such as apples, apricots, cherries, nectarines, peaches, pears, plums, prunes, and watermelons) and vegetables (such as avocados, cauliflower, mushrooms, and snow peas). In addition, they're frequently used in food manufacturing to improve the texture of processed items and to sweeten "sugar-free" beverages, candies, chewing gums, and mints.

Fending Off FODMAPs

The tables through page 24 show which foods are FODMAP-safe (in reasonable portions), which require caution (the maximum suitable serving size will be listed in parentheses), and which foods should be avoided entirely. You can use these tables as guides for both food shopping and meal planning. Please be aware that not every food has been tested for FODMAP content, so these lists aren't all-inclusive; more and more foods are being tested by the Monash University researchers as funding becomes available.

It's important to bear in mind that consuming even recommended quantities of FODMAP-safe foods can be troublesome if too many of these foods are ingested at a single sitting. Note also that some foods are in the "safe" zone when consumed fresh (such as grapes) but are relegated to the "caution" or "danger" zone when dried (such as raisins). That's because FODMAPs become more concentrated in some foods when moisture is removed from them or when the food is subjected to certain manufacturing processes.

TABLE 1 FRUITS AND FRUIT JUICES

SAFE SERVING SIZE = 1 SMALL FRUIT, ½ TO 1 CUP PIECES, OR ¾ CUP BERRIES		CAUTION DON'T EXCEED MAXIMUM AMOUNT LISTED	DANGER AVOID THESE FOODS COMPLETELY	
Banana, firm	Orange	Avocado (⅛ avocado)	Apple, fresh or dried	Grapefruit
Blueberries	Papaya	Banana, ripe (⅓ banana)	Apple juice, fresh or reconstituted	Mango, fresh or dried
Cantaloupe	Passion fruit	Banana chips (10 chips)		Nectarine
Clementine	Pawpaw, fresh	Coconut, shredded dried (¼ cup)	Apricot, fresh or dried	Orange juice, reconstituted
Coconut, fresh (½ cup)	Pineapple, fresh	Cranberries, dried (1 Tbsp)	Apricot juice	
Cranberry juice (1 cup)	Plantain, peeled	Currants (1 Tbsp)	Blackberries	Peach
Dragon fruit	Prickly pear	Longans (5 longans)	Boysenberries	Pear, fresh or dried
Durian	Raspberries, red	Lychees (5 lychees)	Cherries	Persimmon
Grapes	Rhubarb	Orange juice, fresh (½ cup)	Coconut water	Pineapple, dried
Honeydew melon	Star fruit (carambola)	Pawpaw, dried (1 piece)	Custard apple	Plum
Kiwifruit		Pomegranate (¼ cup seeds; ½ small)	Dates	Prunes
Lemon juice (1 tsp)	Strawberries		Figs, fresh or dried	Sultanas
Lime juice (1 tsp)	Tamarind	Raisins (1 Tbsp)	Fruit juice (other than cranberry, lemon, or lime juice)	Tamarillo
Mandarin	Tangelo	Rambutan (2 rambutans)		Tropical blend juice
			Goji berries, dried	Watermelon

Source: Created with data from Monash University, Low FODMAP smartphone app, http://goo.gl/0SmhYb; Monash University, *Low FODMAP Diet for Irritable Bowel Syndrome* (blog), fodmapmonash.blogspot.com; and Sue Shepherd and Peter Gibson, *The Complete Low-FODMAP Diet* (New York: The Experiment, 2013).

TABLE 2 VEGETABLES

SAFE	CAUTION	DANGER
SERVING SIZE = ½ TO 1 CUP UNLESS OTHERWISE NOTED	DON'T EXCEED MAXIMUM AMOUNT LISTED	AVOID THESE FOODS COMPLETELY

SAFE		CAUTION	DANGER
Alfalfa sprouts	Mushrooms, oyster	Artichoke hearts, canned (2 Tbsp)	Artichoke, globe
Arugula	Nori	Beet root (2 slices)	Artichoke, Jerusalem
Bamboo shoots	Okra (6 pods)	Broccoli (½ cup)	Asparagus
Bean sprouts	Olives, black or green	Brussels sprouts (2 sprouts)	Cauliflower
Bell pepper, green	Onion, spring (green tops/leaves only)*	Butternut squash (¼ cup, diced)	Garlic
Bell pepper, red	Parsnip	Cabbage, savoy (½ cup)	Leek bulb
Bok choy	Potato, with peel	Celery (¼ medium stalk)	Mushrooms (except oyster mushrooms)
Cabbage, common green	Radicchio	Corn, sweet (½ cob)	Onion, Spanish
Cabbage, common red	Radishes	Peas, snow (5 pods)	Onion, spring, bulb
Carrot	Rutabaga	Pumpkin, canned (¼ cup)	Onion, white
Celeriac	Sea vegetables	Sweet potato (½ cup or ½ small potato)	Peas, fresh or frozen
Chard/Swiss chard, any variety	Scallion greens (green part only)*	Taro (½ cup, diced)	Peas, sugar snap
Chicory leaves, fresh	Spinach	Tomatoes, sun-dried (2 pieces)	Scallion, bulb
Chile, green or red (1 Tbsp)	Squash, kabocha		Shallots
Chives (1 Tbsp)	Squash, patty pan		
Choy sum	Squash, spaghetti		
Collard greens	Squash, yellow		
Cucumber	Tomato, common		
Eggplant	Tomato, Roma		
Endive	Tomatoes, canned		
Fennel, bulb and leaves	Tomatoes, cherry or grape		
Galangal	Tomatoes, cocktail or Campari		
Gingerroot	Turnip		
Green beans	Water chestnuts		
Kale	Yam		
Leek leaves (green part only)*	Zucchini		
Lettuce, all types			

*Many people with IBS are able to tolerate the green leaves of scallions, leeks, and spring onions (not the white portion or bulbs), but some are not. Assess your own tolerance levels.

Source: Created with data from Monash University, Low FODMAP smartphone app, http://goo.gl/0SmhYb; Monash University, *Low FODMAP Diet for Irritable Bowel Syndrome* (blog), fodmapmonash.blogspot.com; and Sue Shepherd and Peter Gibson, *The Complete Low-FODMAP Diet* (New York: The Experiment, 2013).

TABLE 3 BREADS AND GRAINS

SAFE FOLLOW THE SERVING SIZE LISTED		CAUTION DON'T EXCEED MAXIMUM AMOUNT LISTED	DANGER AVOID THESE FOODS COMPLETELY
Bread, 100% sourdough spelt (2 slices)*	Quinoa, black, red, white (1 cup cooked)	Amaranth puffed cereal (¼ cup)	Amaranth flour
Bread, 100% sourdough wheat (2 slices)*	Quinoa cereal flakes (1 cup)	Bread, 100% sourdough oat (1 slice)	Barley
Bread, gluten-free, plain, vegan (check ingredients; 2 slices)	Quinoa flour (⅔ cup as an ingredient)	Bread, gluten-free, multigrain, vegan (1 slice)	Bran, wheat
Bread, millet (2 slices)	Rice: basmati, brown, white (1 cup cooked)	Rice cereal flakes (¼ cup)	Bread, gluten-free, oat
Buckwheat flour (⅔ cup as an ingredient)	Rice bran (2 tablespoons)	Spelt pasta (½ cup cooked)	Bulgur
Buckwheat groats (¾ cup cooked)	Rice cakes, plain (2 rice cakes)		Couscous
Corn chips, plain (2 ounces)	Rice cereal, puffed or popped (½ cup)		Einkorn
Corn flour (⅔ cup as an ingredient)	Rice crackers, small, plain (20 crackers)		Emmer
Corn Thins (1 Corn Thin)	Rice flour (⅔ cup as an ingredient)		Freekeh
Cornflakes, gluten-free (½ cup)	Seitan (about ⅓ cup)†		Kamut
Cornstarch (⅔ cup as an ingredient)	Sorghum flour (⅔ cup as an ingredient)		Muesli
Millet, hulled (1 cup cooked)	Spelt flour, sieved (⅔ cup as an ingredient)		Rye
Millet flour (⅔ cup as an ingredient)	Tapioca		Wheat (except for 100% sourdough bread, low-FODMAP seitan, or small amounts in prepared foods)*†
Oat bran (2 tablespoons)	Tapioca starch (⅔ cup as an ingredient)		
Oats, quick-cooking (¼ cup dry; ½ cup cooked)	Teff flour (⅔ cup as an ingredient)		
Pasta, gluten-free rice, quinoa, corn (1 cup cooked)	Tortilla chips, plain (1 cup)		
Polenta (1 cup cooked)	Tortillas, brown rice (1 large tortilla)		
Popcorn, plain (1 cup)	Tortillas, corn (2 small)		
Potato chips, plain (1 cup)	Wild rice (1 cup cooked)		
Potato starch (⅔ cup as an ingredient)			

*Many people with IBS are able to tolerate 100% sourdough spelt bread and 100% sourdough wheat bread that is prepared using no yeast (just sourdough cultures) and a long, slow rising time (one to two days). The traditional sourdough process decreases the concentration of FODMAPs and makes the bread more digestible. Assess your own tolerance levels.

†Seitan (vital wheat gluten) is well tolerated by most IBS sufferers because it is pure protein and contains none of the carbohydrates that cause symptoms (as long as no high-FODMAP ingredients are added to it). Seitan should not be consumed by people with celiac disease, gluten intolerance, or wheat allergy.

Source: Created with data from Monash University, Low FODMAP smartphone app, http://goo.gl/0SmhYb; Monash University, *Low FODMAP Diet for Irritable Bowel Syndrome* (blog), fodmapmonash.blogspot.com; and Sue Shepherd and Peter Gibson, *The Complete Low-FODMAP Diet* (New York: The Experiment, 2013).

TABLE 4 NUTS AND SEEDS

SAFE FOLLOW THE SERVING SIZE LISTED		CAUTION DON'T EXCEED MAXIMUM AMOUNT LISTED	DANGER AVOID THESE FOODS COMPLETELY
Brazil nuts (10 nuts)	Pine nuts (1 Tbsp)	Almond butter (1 Tbsp)	Cashews
Chestnuts, boiled (20 nuts)	Poppy seeds, black or white (2 Tbsp)	Almonds (10 nuts)	Pistachios
Chia seeds (2 Tbsp)*	Pumpkin seeds (2 Tbsp)	Flaxseeds (1 Tbsp)	
Macadamia nuts (20 nuts)	Sesame seeds (1 Tbsp)	Hazelnuts (10 nuts)	
Peanut butter (2 Tbsp)	Sunflower seeds (2 tsp)	Tahini (1 Tbsp)	
Peanuts (32 nuts)	Walnuts (10 halves)		
Pecans (10 halves)			

*Monash University reports that although chia seeds have tested low for FOD-MAPs, anecdotal evidence indicates that some people with IBS do not tolerate chia seeds well. Assess your own tolerance levels.

Source: Created with data from Monash University, Low FODMAP smartphone app, http://goo.gl/0SmhYb; Monash University, *Low FODMAP Diet for Irritable Bowel Syndrome* (blog), fodmapmonash.blogspot.com; and Sue Shepherd and Peter Gibson, *The Complete Low-FODMAP Diet* (New York: The Experiment, 2013).

TABLE 5 LEGUMES*

SAFE FOLLOW THE SERVING SIZE LISTED	CAUTION DON'T EXCEED MAXIMUM AMOUNT LISTED	DANGER AVOID THESE FOODS COMPLETELY
Chana dal, boiled (½ cup cooked)	Butter beans, canned, rinsed well (¼ cup)	Baked beans
Lentils, canned, rinsed well (½ cup)	Chickpeas, canned, rinsed well (¼ cup)	Black beans
Miso, chickpea or soy (1 Tbsp)	Lentils, green, boiled (¼ cup cooked)	Borlotti beans
Tempeh, plain (1 slice; 3.5 ounces)	Lentils, red, boiled (¼ cup cooked)	Broad beans
Tofu, plain, firm (⅔ cup cubed; 6 ounces)	Lima beans, boiled (¼ cup cooked)	Hummus
Urid dal, boiled (½ cup cooked)	Mung beans, boiled (¼ cup cooked)	Kidney beans, red or white
		Peas, fresh or frozen
		Soybeans
		Split peas
		Tofu, silken

*Canned lentils and chickpeas will have lower amounts of FODMAPs than those cooked from dried beans. The fermentation process that tempeh undergoes helps reduce the amount of FODMAPs in the beans, making it more digestible. Firm tofu (not soft or silken tofu) is acceptable because the majority of FODMAPs are drained off during the tofu-making process. Miso is acceptable on a low-FODMAP diet because of how it is processed.

Source: Created with data from Monash University, Low FODMAP smartphone app, http://goo.gl/0SmhYb; Monash University, *Low FODMAP Diet for Irritable Bowel Syndrome* (blog), fodmapmonash.blogspot.com; and Sue Shepherd and Peter Gibson, *The Complete Low-FODMAP Diet* (New York: The Experiment, 2013).

TABLE 6 SWEETENERS, CONFECTIONS, AND OILS

SAFE FOLLOW THE SERVING SIZE LISTED		CAUTION DON'T EXCEED MAXIMUM AMOUNT LISTED	DANGER AVOID THESE FOODS COMPLETELY
Cacao powder (2 heaping tsp) Chocolate, dark (5 squares; 1 ounce) Cocoa powder (2 heaping tsp) Jam, strawberry or raspberry (2 Tbsp)	Maple syrup (2 Tbsp) Marmalade, orange (2 Tbsp) Oil, all types (1 Tbsp) Rice syrup (1 Tbsp) Stevia, powder (2 sachets) Sugar, brown, palm, raw, white (1 Tbsp)	Carob powder (1 heaping tsp)	Agave nectar Artificial sweeteners Fruit bars Granola bars

Source: Created with data from Monash University, Low FODMAP smartphone app, http://goo.gl/0SmhYb; Monash University, *Low FODMAP Diet for Irritable Bowel Syndrome* (blog), fodmapmonash.blogspot.com; and Sue Shepherd and Peter Gibson, *The Complete Low-FODMAP Diet* (New York: The Experiment, 2013).

TABLE 7 CONDIMENTS AND SEASONINGS

SAFE FOLLOW THE SERVING SIZE LISTED		DANGER AVOID THESE FOODS COMPLETELY
Asafetida (¼ tsp) Capers (1 Tbsp) Herbs: basil, cilantro, dill, oregano, parsley, rosemary, sage, spearmint, tarragon, thyme (1 cup fresh; ¼ cup dried) Miso, chickpea or soy (1 Tbsp)* Mustard, Dijon (1 Tbsp) Mustard, yellow (1 Tbsp)†	Nutritional yeast flakes (2 Tbsp) Spices, ground: allspice, black pepper, cayenne, cinnamon, cloves, coriander seeds, cumin, curry powder, dry mustard, fennel seeds, fenugreek seeds, five spice, ginger, mustard seeds, nutmeg, paprika, saffron, star anise, turmeric (1 tsp) Tamari or soy sauce (2 Tbsp) Tamarind paste (1½ tsp) Vinegar, balsamic (1 Tbsp) Vinegar, cider (2 Tbsp) Vinegar, rice (2 Tbsp) Wasabi (1 tsp)	Pasta sauce, with onion and/or garlic Pesto with garlic Pickles and relish with garlic and/or onion

*Miso is acceptable on a low-FODMAP diet because of how it is processed.

†Read the label carefully to be sure that no onion, garlic, or other high-FODMAP ingredients have been added.

Source: Created with data from Monash University, Low FODMAP smartphone app, http://goo.gl/0SmhYb; Monash University, *Low FODMAP Diet for Irritable Bowel Syndrome* (blog), fodmapmonash.blogspot.com; and Sue Shepherd and Peter Gibson, *The Complete Low-FODMAP Diet* (New York: The Experiment, 2013).

TABLE 8 BEVERAGES

SAFE	CAUTION	DANGER
FOLLOW THE SERVING SIZE LISTED	DON'T EXCEED MAXIMUM AMOUNT LISTED	AVOID THESE FOODS COMPLETELY

SAFE		CAUTION	DANGER
Almond milk (1 cup)	Hemp milk (1 cup)	Coconut milk beverage (½ cup)	Apple juice
Beer (1 standard can)*	Rice milk (1 cup)	Tea, chai, weak (1 cup)	Coconut water, fresh
Gin (1 ounce)*	Soymilk, made only with soy protein isolate or extract (1 cup)	Tea, dandelion (½ cup)	Coconut water, packaged
Cocoa, sweetened, powder (2 heaping tsp)			Oat milk
Coconut milk, canned (½ cup)	Tea, decaf or regular: black, ginger, green, peppermint, or white (1 cup)		Orange juice (fresh or reconstituted)
Coffee, decaf or regular: black or with low-FODMAP nondairy milk (1 cup)	Vegetable blend juice: tomato-based, no onion or garlic (1 cup)		Soymilk (made with whole soybeans)
Cranberry juice (1 cup)	Vodka (1 ounce)*		Rum
Drinking chocolate, powder (2 heaping tsp)	Whiskey (1 ounce)*		Tea, chai, strong
Espresso, decaf or regular: black or with low-FODMAP nondairy milk (single shot)	Wine: red, white, or sparkling (1 glass)*		Tea, chamomile
			Tea, fennel
			Tea, oolong
			Wine, low-glycemic index
			Wine, sticky

*Alcohol is an irritant to the digestive tract. Have only a limited amount and always consume alcohol with food.

Source: Created with data from Monash University, Low FODMAP smartphone app, http://goo.gl/0SmhYb; Monash University, *Low FODMAP Diet for Irritable Bowel Syndrome* (blog), fodmapmonash.blogspot.com; and Sue Shepherd and Peter Gibson, *The Complete Low-FODMAP Diet* (New York: The Experiment, 2013).

Navigating FODMAPs Safely

4

Because FODMAPs are found almost exclusively in plant foods, it can seem daunting if not impossible for vegans with IBS to have a well-balanced, low-FODMAP eating plan. Vegans in general are routinely, although unjustifiably, questioned about whether they're getting enough protein, but these concerns become disproportionately magnified in light of a low-FODMAP diet. That's because most beans, a primary plant-based protein source, aren't generally well tolerated by people with IBS and are therefore very limited on a low-FODMAP regimen.

Fortunately, all plant foods (except alcohol, oil, and sugar) contain at least a modicum of protein, so as long as you're eating a sufficient amount of whole, fresh foods (rather than sugary, refined, or high-fat processed foods), protein shouldn't be an issue. In addition, there are plenty of well-tolerated, low-FODMAP, plant-based sources of concentrated proteins—such as lentils (in limited quantities), chickpeas (in limited quantities), tofu, tempeh, seitan, quinoa, peanuts and peanut butter, and most (but not all) nuts and seeds—which should put to rest any lingering worries.

Here are a few more pointers regarding vegan culinary options:

Legumes, legume flours, and miso. As noted above, most legumes (beans, lentils, and peas) are extremely high in FODMAPs and aren't well tolerated by most people with IBS. The two exceptions are regulated amounts of canned chickpeas (no more than ¼ cup) and canned lentils (no more than ½ cup). Canned chickpeas and lentils have fewer FODMAPs than other legumes, including dried chickpeas and dried lentils. To further remove FODMAPs, always drain and rinse canned chickpeas and lentils thoroughly before using, as additional FODMAPs lurk in the liquid.

Legume flours (chickpea flour, lentil flour, pea flour, and soy flour) in modest proportions as ingredients in packaged products or recipes are considered acceptable and shouldn't trigger symptoms in most people with IBS. Miso made from chickpeas or soybeans is generally well tolerated in reasonable amounts because the fermentation process used to make these products consumes a fair portion of the FODMAPs.

Nuts and seeds. Nuts and seeds and their butters are tasty, multipurpose sources of concentrated plant protein. However, they're also high in fat (a common IBS trigger). In addition, the amount of FODMAPs ingested can slip into the danger zone if nuts or seeds are consumed in quantities greater than recommended. Keep serving sizes to no larger than 2 teaspoons to 2 tablespoons (see page 22 for specific amounts per nut or seed) and limit other high-FODMAP foods at the same meal.

Sourdough spelt or sourdough wheat bread. A number of people with IBS are able to tolerate 100% sourdough spelt bread and 100% sourdough wheat bread (white or whole wheat) that is prepared using no yeast and involves a long, slow rising time (one to two days). That's because this traditional sourdough process decreases the concentration of FODMAPs, resulting in breads that are more digestible. Making 100% sourdough bread is very time-consuming, however, and just a few commercial bakeries in North America offer it. In addition, the FODMAP content of these breads may vary depending on the sourdough fermentation method used by the bakery and whether any high-FODMAP ingredients are added, so do a trial of one to two slices with a meal to assess your tolerance.

Check your natural food store's freezer section (that's where this bread is usually kept) and read the ingredient label carefully or contact the bakery directly to verify that they use a long, slow leavening process and that their bread contains nothing other than spelt flour or wheat flour, sourdough cultures, and salt. Because spelt is a relative of wheat and contains gluten, it should not be consumed by anyone with celiac disease, gluten intolerance, or wheat allergy.

Soymilk, soy cheese, soy creamer, and soy yogurt. When soymilk, soy cheese, soy creamer, and soy yogurt are made with soy protein isolate or soy extract, not whole soybeans, they are considered low-FODMAP foods. Read labels closely or contact the manufacturer to ensure the product is made only from soy protein isolate or extract (not from the whole beans) and that no high-FODMAP ingredients have been added. Almond milk (see page 46 for a homemade version) and hemp milk should also be well tolerated, as should almond-milk yogurt and coconut-milk yogurt (check ingredients of individual brands and flavors). Choose fortified or enriched products whenever possible.

Rice milk was previously believed to be high in FODMAPs when Monash University originally tested it in 2015. However, further research showed that rice milk is actually low in FODMAPs for a one-cup serving. The confusion occurred with the initial testing because of the enzymes used in the processing of rice milk. The enzymes don't fully break down the starch in the rice, so small amounts of oligosaccharides are left behind. However, not all oligosaccharides are malabsorbed like fructans and GOS. In fact, some types of starch-derived oligosaccharides are digestible, and it was these digestible oligosaccharides that were getting mixed in with the fructans and GOS during the original FODMAP testing, resulting in a false high-FODMAP reading. Monash University has since developed new testing protocols that separate out the different types of oligosaccharides to provide more accurate results.

Tempeh. Tempeh is made from fermented soybeans and is low in FODMAPs because of how it's processed. As long as it doesn't contain added high-FODMAP seasonings and portions are reasonably sized (see page 22), tempeh should be well tolerated by most people with IBS. Note that some tempeh contains wheat (usually in the form of soy sauce) or barley, so if you have celiac disease, gluten intolerance, or wheat allergy, be sure to read the product label carefully.

Tofu. Plain superfirm and extra-firm tofu are generally well tolerated (see box, page 28) on a low-FODMAP diet. These types of tofu are devoid of the carbohydrates that cause IBS symptoms, as long as they aren't seasoned with high-FODMAP ingredients. However, avoid softer varieties of tofu, including silken tofu, as these retain more of the bean's natural indigestible carbohydrates.

Wheat, Gluten, Seitan, and the Low-FODMAP Diet

A low-FODMAP diet isn't a gluten-free diet. The only people with IBS who need to avoid gluten and gluten-containing products are those who have celiac disease, gluten intolerance, or wheat allergy. For everyone else, wheat is only problematic when it's the main part of carbohydrate-based foods, such as breads (other than 100% sourdough spelt or wheat breads), cakes and other baked goods, cereals, or pastas. Foods that contain very minimal amounts of wheat, such as soy sauce or even light breading on vegetables, shouldn't cause symptoms for most people with IBS.

Wheat derivatives that don't contain fructans are also safe on a low-FODMAP diet. These include caramel coloring, dextrin, dextrose, maltodextrin, and wheat starch, all of which are frequently used in food manufacturing and are free of FODMAPs.

Seitan is pure protein made from the gluten extracted from wheat (also known as vital wheat gluten) and is carbohydrate-free. As long as the seitan doesn't contain added high-FODMAP ingredients or seasonings, such as garlic or onion, it should be a well-tolerated food for most vegans with IBS. In addition, seitan is an excellent source of concentrated protein and can be used in a wide range of savory dishes. Be aware that some brands of seitan contain whole legumes and/or legume flours, so

The less liquid that's in tofu, the firmer the tofu will be and the fewer FODMAPs it will contain. Superfirm tofu is the best choice, especially the kind that's vacuum sealed and not packed in water, as it will be quite dense straight out of the package. Any tofu that's packed in water will be softer and will contain slightly more FODMAPs. It also won't be as meaty in recipes. If you're unable to obtain vacuum-packed superfirm tofu in your local stores, or even if you are but you want the ultimate in firm tofu, you can press superfirm or extra-firm tofu to get an incredibly dense and meaty texture (which I highly recommend doing).

The easiest, fastest, and tidiest way to press tofu is to use a tofu press. A press will also provide consistent commercial-quality outcomes, resulting in the firmest tofu possible in just about thirty minutes. Although tofu presses may seem pricey, they are a one-time investment that will be well worth the expense, especially if you use tofu frequently. My favorite press is the TofuXpress (tofuxpress.com), because it produces evenly pressed, ultrafirm tofu cleanly, quickly, evenly, and reliably. Plus, the whole caboodle (tofu and press) can be conveniently put in the refrigerator, so you can press the tofu for hours, if you like, to create the densest, most delicious tofu imaginable.

If you prefer to press tofu without a tofu press, it will be a little messy and will take longer to achieve somewhat similar (though not quite as firm) results. But if you still insist, here's how to do it:

1. Slice open the package and drain the water. Rinse the tofu and pat it dry.

2. Put a thick, clean tea towel or several layers of paper towels on a rimmed baking sheet or plate.

3. Put the tofu on the towel. Put another thick, clean tea towel or several layers of paper towels on top of it.

4. Put an inverted rimmed baking sheet or plate on top of the towel.

5. Put one or more heavy objects, such as large books or canned goods, on top.

6. Let the tofu rest for at least 30 minutes. The longer the tofu is pressed, the firmer it will be. If you want to press it longer than 30 minutes, move the entire setup to the refrigerator. Drain off the liquid that accumulates as the tofu is being pressed and replace the tea towels and paper towels as needed when they become saturated.

read labels closely if you are supersensitive to these ingredients. Although chickpea flour, lentil flour, and pea flour are high-FODMAP foods, as long as they're used in small amounts as ingredients (see Reading Food Labels, page 31), they shouldn't cause symptoms in most people with IBS. Assess your own tolerance level or seek out seitan that is free of these and other high-FODMAP ingredients. Note that although vital wheat gluten is a common component of commercial veggie burgers and vegan meat alternatives, these prepared products generally also contain garlic, legumes, onion, wheat flour, and other high-FODMAP ingredients that are poorly tolerated and therefore aren't suitable on a low-FODMAP diet.

Onion and Garlic

Onion is one of the most concentrated sources of FODMAPs and should be avoided, even in minute amounts, if you're following a strict low-FODMAP diet. Onion isn't considered an allergen, so manufacturers aren't required to declare it on product labels. And to complicate matters, onion is one of the most ubiquitous ingredients and therefore among the most difficult to avoid. If you request the ingredient list of prepared vegan foods at your natural food store, read the labels of products in the refrigerated and frozen-food aisles, ask for detailed ingredients of menu items at your local vegan restaurant, or inquire about ingredients at a vegan potluck, you'll be hard pressed to find anything that doesn't contain onion. It's nearly impossible to find a savory vegan product, prepared food, frozen food, restaurant option, or recipe that doesn't contain onion in some form. Even if onion isn't directly listed, it may be a "hidden" ingredient as a component of another seasoning, such as chile powder, all-purpose seasoning, or a spice blend. Onion is almost always an ingredient in vegan soups, sauces, gravies, and marinades, and it's commonly used in frozen potatoes, vegan cheeses, vegan dips, faux meats, veggie burgers, seasoned tofu and seitan, tempeh bacon, packaged vegetable broths, and veggie bouillon cubes. Be aware that "onion" refers to any member of the onion family, regardless of its type or form. This includes onion, onion powder, shallots, leeks, and the white part (bulb) of scallions. Although most people with IBS can tolerate the green part (leaves) of scallions and leeks, you will need to assess your own tolerance levels.

Garlic is equally as prevalent as onion and is also extremely high in FODMAPs. While some IBS sufferers can withstand tiny amounts of garlic in prepared foods, many cannot. Again, you will need to test your own tolerance levels. Alternatives to onion and garlic include chives (fresh or freeze-dried), fresh and dried herbs, spices (see page 23), and garlic-infused olive oil, which is readily available in supermarkets, natural food stores, and online (see Resources, page 133). Garlic-infused oil is free of FODMAPs, highly flavorful, and very convenient. Onion-infused and shallot-infused oils are also free of FODMAPs and a boon to low-FODMAP cooking, but they're more difficult to find in North America. Making infused oils with garlic, onion, or shallots at home isn't recommended because of the high risk of botulism (which is not a concern with commercial products).

Asafetida, also known as hing, is an Indian seasoning with a fetid aroma and unique flavor that tastes very similar to onion and garlic, especially when it's cooked briefly in hot oil. Look for it in Indian spice shops. Many brands of asafetida contain a small amount of wheat flour; if this is a concern for you, seek out brands that are gluten-free and contain rice flour instead (see Resources, page 133). Just a pinch of asafetida goes a long way in cooking, so a small jar should last you quite a while.

TABLE 9 COMMON HIGH-FODMAP INGREDIENTS AND POTENTIAL SOURCES

INGREDIENT	POTENTIAL SOURCES
Chicory	Coffee alternatives, vegan yogurts
Fructan	High-fiber foods
Fructooligosaccharides (FOS)	Protein powders, sports drinks, sports gels
Fructose	Cakes, confections, soft drinks, sports drinks, sports gels
Fruit juice (such as apple or pear juice)	Beverage blends, breakfast cereals, granola bars, vegan yogurts
Fruit pieces (such as dates, dried apple, mango, raisins, etc.) as a significant portion of the food	Breakfast cereals, granola bars, smoothies, vegan yogurts
Garlic, garlic powder, garlic salt	Crackers, dips, flavored chips and snack foods, hummus, meat alternatives, pasta sauces, prepared foods, salad dressings, soups, vegan cheeses, vegetable bouillon cubes, vegetable broths, vegetable stocks, veggie burgers, veggie dogs, veggie sausages
High-fructose corn syrup	Breads, granola bars, jams, soft drinks
Inulin	Breads, crackers, vegan yogurts
Isomalt	Chewing gums, mints
Mannitol	Artificially sweetened beverages, candies, chewing gums, cough medicines, lozenges, mints
Onion, onion powder, onion salt	Crackers, dips, flavored chips and snack foods, meat alternatives, pasta sauces, prepared foods, salad dressings, soups, vegan cheeses, vegetable bouillon cubes, vegetable broths, vegetable stocks, veggie burgers, veggie dogs, veggie sausages
Rye	Breads, breakfast cereals, crackers
Sorbitol	Artificially sweetened beverages, candies, chewing gums, cough medicines, lozenges, mints
Wheat as a main ingredient (listed first to third on the ingredient list)	Breads, breakfast cereals, crackers, pastas
Xylitol	Artificially sweetened beverages, candies, chewing gums, cough medicines, lozenges, mints

Reading Food Labels

As noted earlier, FODMAPs are only problematic when they're consumed in measurable quantities. Foods with tiny amounts of FODMAPs don't usually cause IBS symptoms. The US Food and Drug Administration's labeling guidelines for food manufacturers require that product labels list ingredients in descending order of predominance by weight, which means that the first ingredient listed is in the highest quantity and the last ingredient listed is in the lowest quantity. If an ingredient is present in small amounts or is near the end of a lengthy ingredient list, it should be safe to consume. When you start to reintroduce higher-FODMAP foods (see page 38), you may want to try products that contain high-FODMAP ingredients, such as garlic powder, when they're listed as minor players. You can then monitor your tolerance of them.

Learning how to read food labels can assist you with recognizing suitable low-FODMAP foods. Be aware, however, that it's not always possible to identify high-FODMAP ingredients. Some foods that appear to be low in FODMAPs may not be. So even if you find a product that looks like it should be safe, do a test trial to confirm that you're able to tolerate it.

Table 9 (page 30) contains a list of some common FODMAP-containing ingredients and products in which they are often found. Note that this table is not exhaustive and not all products listed will necessarily contain these ingredients. Always check food labels to see the specific ingredients the product contains.

Dining Out

Although following a low-FODMAP vegan diet may seem daunting at first, as time passes and you become more familiar with what you can and can't tolerate, you'll also become more comfortable planning meals and cooking. Dining at restaurants or at the homes of family members or friends can be more challenging, however, because you can't always control what you're being served. If you're less strict with the diet when you're away from home, you might suffer more symptoms for a few days. Although socializing is important, it's also essential to feel safe when eating out and not have to worry about how you're going to feel afterward.

At Restaurants

Fortunately, most vegan restaurants that prepare food to order can easily customize dishes for you. And because there is a growing number of people with food intolerances, even the staff at many mainstream restaurants have become accustomed to answering questions about their ingredients, so you needn't feel timid. The low-FODMAP diet isn't a gluten-free diet, but restaurants that offer gluten-free options will likely have a greater selection and be more willing and better equipped to modify dishes so they're both vegan and IBS-friendly. Here are a few tips that will help make your dining-out experience more enjoyable:

- Write a short summary on a small, wallet-sized card of your dietary needs. It's helpful to not just include what you can't have (garlic, legumes, onion, wheat) but also what you can have (bok choy, carrots, eggplant, green beans, herbs, kale, olive oil, olives, potatoes, rice, rice noodles, soy sauce, spices, spinach, tempeh, tofu, tomatoes, walnuts, zucchini). This will give the chef a starting point for preparing a custom-designed dish you'll love (and one that will love you back).

- Call in advance whenever possible to ensure something suitable will be available for you or that something can be prepared that meets your needs.

- Know that small amounts of wheat in the form of bread crumbs on vegetables or croutons in a salad are generally tolerated by most people with IBS.

- Wheat as an ingredient in sauces, such as soy sauce or a stir-fry sauce, is acceptable on the low-FODMAP diet.

- Tofu and tempeh are good main-dish choices at vegan restaurants, but ask for them to be prepared without onion (including shallots or leeks) or garlic. If scallions are used, make certain the staff understands that only the greens (not the white bulb) should be in the dish.

- Vegan sushi is usually available at Japanese restaurants and is a good choice when made with tofu rather than avocado. Vegan pad thai at Thai restaurants is another welcome option (check that it contains no onion or scallion bulbs), as is a custom-made vegetable stir-fry with rice or rice noodles, which should be available at most Asian restaurants. Mainstream restaurants should be able to provide a baked potato (with olive oil) and a salad (ask for no onions!) with lemon juice or balsamic vinegar and olive oil.

- Avoid soups, gravies, and premade salad dressings unless you're able to obtain a full ingredient list and can be certain of what they contain. If you're comfortable doing so, take your own low-FODMAP vegan dressing, sauce, or gluten-free pasta to the restaurant.

At Friends' Homes

It would be helpful to provide friends and family members with information about the low-FODMAP vegan diet before you go to their homes for a meal. If they already understand a vegan diet, they're one step ahead of the game, but a low-FODMAP diet takes the learning curve to another level. Be patient and try to educate them. Give them a copy of this book. Make a copy of your restaurant card (see above) for them. Ask in advance what they'll be preparing and inquire about any modifications that could be made. Provide some recipes or menu ideas. Offer to bring a low-FODMAP vegan dish that everyone can share. If necessary, eat before you go if you have any concerns about the menu, and nibble on any available safe foods while you're there.

What to Eat When You Can't Eat Anything

When you're in the midst of a flare-up, all food looks like the enemy. Minimizing solid-food intake during this time and consuming only soft and/or well-cooked, low-fiber, low-fat, bland, low-FODMAP choices will help soothe an irritable gut. Depending on whether diarrhea or constipation predominates, here are some options to consider:

- Almond-milk yogurt (check ingredients of various brands and flavors)

- Baked potato (minus the skin)

- Basmati Rice Pudding (page 69), without dried cranberries or nuts

- Coconut-milk yogurt (check ingredients of various brands and flavors)

- Cream of rice hot cereal

- Ginger or peppermint tea

- Gluten-free vegan toast

- Maple-Vanilla Soft Serve (page 72)

- Mashed potatoes

- Peanut Butter–Banana Instant Breakfast Drink (page 73)

- Plain rice cakes or crackers

- Polenta, plain

- Pumpkin Pie Mousse (page 70)

- Rice noodles

- Vanilla Tapioca Pudding (page 68)

- Vegetable broth or stock (low-FODMAP; see page 58), plain or with rice noodles

- Water with a squeeze of lemon

- Well-cooked white rice

Once the worst has passed, it's essential to get back on track as quickly as possible with a more balanced diet. Adding back a variety of low-FODMAP vegetables, fruits, and grains as tolerated will help you to avoid nutrient deficiencies and weight loss.

Table 10 (below) lists many common high-FODMAP foods and suitable low-FODMAP alternatives. This is a good place to start when sorting out what to eat. Take a look at the list of options in the right column and see what appeals to you. Often what sounds good on paper will feel good in your tummy.

TABLE 10 COMMON HIGH-FODMAP FOODS AND LOW-FODMAP ALTERNATIVES

HUNGRY? THIRSTY?	INSTEAD OF HIGH-FODMAP FOODS	CHOOSE LOW-FODMAP ALTERNATIVES
Beverages	apple, pear, and mango juices; chicory-based coffee alternatives	water; juice from low-FODMAP fruits (no more than ½ cup per serving); black tea (no more than 1 cup per day); coffee (no more than 1 cup per day); low-FODMAP herbal tea (ginger or peppermint); low-FODMAP smoothies (see pages 73 and 76)
Breads, Cakes, and Cookies	bread crumbs; bagels; flour tortillas; pita bread; wheat breads; wheat-based cakes, cookies, muffins	brown rice tortillas; corn flake crumbs; corn tortillas and taco shells; gluten-free vegan bread; gluten-free vegan bread crumbs; gluten-free vegan cakes; gluten-free-vegan cookies; gluten-free vegan muffins; 100% sourdough spelt bread or wheat bread (if tolerated); rice cakes, plain; rice crackers, plain; romaine lettuce leaves (instead of sandwich bread)
Cereals	breakfast cereal (wheat-based and/or fruit-sweetened varieties); muesli	Breakfast Quinoa (page 64); cornflakes; cream of rice cereal; quinoa flakes; rice cereal, puffed or popped (no more than ½ cup); rice cereal flakes (no more than ¼ cup); rolled oats (no more than ¼ cup dry); other gluten-free cereals (check ingredients)
Condiments and Spreads	most commercial bouillon cubes, chutneys, dressings, pickles, relishes, sauces, and vegetable broths/stocks contain onion and/or garlic	Bragg Liquid Aminos; hot sauce; miso; mustard; nutritional yeast; orange marmalade; Tabasco; raspberry jam; soy sauce; strawberry jam; tamari; vegan butter); vegan mayo; vinegar (also see Low-FODMAP Staples, pages 45 to 62)
Fats and Oils	applesauce as an oil replacer in baked goods	banana, ripe, mashed; coconut oil; kabocha squash, cooked and mashed; olive oil or other oil; vegan butter (check ingredients)

TABLE 10 (CONTINUED)

HUNGRY? THIRSTY?	INSTEAD OF HIGH-FODMAP FOODS	CHOOSE LOW-FODMAP ALTERNATIVES
Fruits	apple; apricot; Asian pear; avocado; blackberries; boysenberries; cherries; figs; grapefruit; mango; nectarine; peach; pear; persimmon; plum; prunes; watermelon	banana, firm; blueberries; cantaloupe; cranberries; durian; grapes; honeydew melon; kiwifruit; lemon; lime; mandarin; orange; papaya; raspberries; star fruit; strawberries; tangelo; tangerine; tomato
Garlic and Onion	garlic; green onions; leek; ramps; scallions with bulb; shallots	asafetida (hing); chives (fresh or dried); FODMAP-free spices; garlic-infused oil; ginger, fresh or dried; herbs, fresh or dried; leek greens (green leaves only, if tolerated); onion- or shallot-infused oil; scallion greens (green leaves only)
Grains, Grain Flours, and Legume Flours	barley; bulgur; chickpea flour;* couscous; Kamut; lentil flour;* pea flour;* rye; semolina; soy flour;* triticale; wheat bran; wheat flour; wheat germ	arrowroot starch; buckwheat; cornmeal; cornstarch; gluten-free all-purpose flour blends;* millet, hulled; oat bran; oats; polenta; popcorn; potato flour; quinoa; rice (basmati, brown, white); rice bran; rice flour; sago; sorghum; spelt flour, sieved (⅔ cup as an ingredient, if tolerated); tapioca; wild rice
Meat Alternatives	veggie bacon; veggie burgers; veggie chicken; veggie sausage	Chickenless Chicken (page 52); low-FODMAP seitan; tempeh, plain; textured vegetable protein; tofu, firm, plain; Tofu Bacon Strips or Slabs (page 49)
Nuts and Seeds	cashews; pistachios	small amounts of most other nuts or seeds and their butters (see page 22 for portion sizes)
Pasta and Noodles	gnocchi; wheat noodles; wheat pasta	glass noodles; gluten-free, low-FODMAP pasta (corn, quinoa, or rice); 100% buckwheat soba noodles (wheat-free); rice noodles; rice vermicelli
Sweeteners	agave nectar; applesauce; dates; fruit juice concentrate	cane sugar (brown sugar, confectioners' sugar, palm sugar, raw sugar, unbleached cane sugar); maple syrup; molasses; rice syrup; stevia

*These foods contain FODMAPs, but in small amounts as part of a recipe or product ingredient they shouldn't cause IBS symptoms in most people. Assess your own tolerance levels.

Shopping for Gut-Friendly Foods

Although you might think there is little to eat that you can tolerate and that a low-FODMAP vegan diet is overly restrictive, when you take a look at the shopping guide that follows, you'll see there are numerous options from which you can choose. The list is broken down by food category, so you can consider at a glance what to buy, depending on your preferences and what's in season. Print out a copy of the list and use it each week, checking off the items you want to purchase. It will make going to the store a pleasure, and you'll be pleasantly surprised how quickly your cart will be overflowing with delicious, wholesome, tummy-friendly vegan foods.

GUT-FRIENDLY SHOPPING LIST AND PANTRY GUIDE

BREADS AND GRAINS

- ○ Bread, gluten-free, vegan (check ingredients)
- ○ Bread, 100% sourdough spelt
- ○ Bread, 100% sourdough wheat
- ○ Buckwheat groats
- ○ Corn chips, plain
- ○ Corn flake crumbs
- ○ Corn Thins

- ○ Cornflakes, gluten-free
- ○ Crispy rice cereal
- ○ Glass noodles
- ○ Gluten-free cereal (check ingredients)
- ○ Millet, hulled
- ○ Oats, rolled, quick-cooking
- ○ Pasta, gluten-free
- ○ Pasta, quinoa
- ○ Pasta, rice

- ○ Polenta (coarse cornmeal)
- ○ Popcorn, plain
- ○ Puffed rice cereal
- ○ Quinoa (all colors)
- ○ Rice, arborio
- ○ Rice, basmati
- ○ Rice, brown
- ○ Rice, flakes
- ○ Rice, white

- ○ Rice cakes, plain
- ○ Rice crackers, plain
- ○ Rice noodles
- ○ Seitan (check ingredients)
- ○ Tapioca pearls, small
- ○ Tortilla chips, plain
- ○ Tortillas, brown rice
- ○ Tortillas, corn
- ○ Wild rice

NUTS AND SEEDS

- ○ Almond butter
- ○ Almonds
- ○ Brazil nuts
- ○ Chestnuts
- ○ Chia seeds (any color)

- ○ Flaxseeds (any color)
- ○ Hazelnuts
- ○ Macadamia nuts
- ○ Peanut butter
- ○ Peanut butter powder

- ○ Peanut flour
- ○ Peanuts
- ○ Pecans
- ○ Pine nuts
- ○ Poppy seeds (any color)

- ○ Pumpkin seeds
- ○ Sesame seeds
- ○ Sunflower seeds
- ○ Tahini
- ○ Walnuts

FRUITS

- ○ Banana
- ○ Blueberries, fresh and frozen
- ○ Breadfruit
- ○ Cantaloupe
- ○ Clementine
- ○ Prickly pear
- ○ Coconut

- ○ Dragon fruit
- ○ Durian
- ○ Grapes (seedless; all types)
- ○ Honeydew melon
- ○ Kiwifruit
- ○ Lemon
- ○ Lime

- ○ Mandarin
- ○ Orange, navel
- ○ Papaya
- ○ Passion fruit
- ○ Pawpaw, fresh
- ○ Pineapple, fresh, frozen, and canned in juice
- ○ Plantain

- ○ Raspberries, red
- ○ Rhubarb
- ○ Star fruit
- ○ Strawberries, fresh and frozen
- ○ Tangelo

VEGETABLES

- Alfalfa sprouts
- Arugula
- Bamboo shoots
- Basil
- Bean sprouts
- Bell pepper (all colors)
- Bok choy
- Broccoli, fresh and frozen
- Cabbage, common green
- Cabbage, common red
- Carrot
- Celeriac
- Chard/Swiss chard
- Chicory leaves
- Chiles (red and green)
- Chives
- Choy sum
- Cilantro
- Collard greens
- Cucumber
- Eggplant
- Endive
- Fennel bulb
- Fennel leaves
- Gai lan
- Galangal
- Gingerroot
- Green beans
- Kale (all kinds)
- Leek (leaves only)
- Lettuce (all kinds)
- Mesclun
- Nori
- Okra
- Olives, black or green
- Parsley, flat-leaf
- Parsnip
- Potato
- Pumpkin, canned
- Radicchio
- Radish
- Rutabaga
- Scallions (green part only)
- Spinach, baby
- Squash, kabocha
- Squash, patty pan
- Squash, spaghetti
- Squash, yellow
- Tomato (all types), fresh and canned
- Turnip
- Turnip greens
- Water chestnuts
- Yam (not sweet potato)
- Zucchini

SEASONINGS AND SWEETENERS

- Asafetida (hing)
- Bragg Liquid Aminos
- Ginger, fresh or jarred
- Herbs, fresh and dried (basil, bay leaves, chives, cilantro, coriander, dill weed, lemongrass, marjoram, oregano, parsley, rosemary, sage, spearmint, tarragon, thyme)
- Liquid smoke
- Maple syrup, pure
- Miso (chickpea and light)
- Mustard, Dijon
- Mustard, stoneground
- Mustard, yellow
- Nutritional yeast flakes
- Rice syrup
- Sea salt
- Soy sauce
- Stevia
- Spices, dried or ground (allspice, bay leaves, black pepper, cardamom, cayenne, cloves, cinnamon, coriander, cumin, curry powder, dry mustard, fennel seeds, fenugreek seeds, five spice, ginger, mustard seeds, nutmeg, paprika, poppy seeds, smoked paprika, turmeric)
- Tamari
- Sugar, brown
- Sugar, palm
- Sugar, unbleached cane
- Tabasco
- Tamari
- Vanilla extract
- Vinegar, balsamic
- Vinegar, champagne
- Vinegar, cider
- Vinegar, rice
- Vinegar, wine (red and white)

BEVERAGES, OILS, AND OTHER PANTRY STAPLES

- Alcohol (beer, gin, vodka, whiskey, wine)
- Butter, vegan
- Capers
- Chickpeas, canned
- Chocolate, dark
- Chocolate chips, dark
- Chocolate chips, mini
- Cocoa powder, unsweetened
- Coconut, unsweetened shredded dried
- Coconut milk, light
- Jam, raspberry
- Jam, strawberry
- Lecithin, sunflower liquid
- Lentils, canned
- Marmalade, orange
- Mayonnaise, vegan
- Nondairy milk (almond, hemp, quinoa)
- Oil, basil-infused
- Oil, coconut
- Oil, extra-virgin olive
- Oil, garlic-infused
- Oil, herb-infused
- Oil, lemon-infused
- Oil, onion- or shallot-infused
- Oil, safflower
- Tea (black, ginger, green, peppermint, white)
- Tempeh, plain
- Tofu, extra-firm
- Tofu, superfirm
- Tomato purée
- Tomatoes, canned (diced, crushed, fire-roasted, whole)

Reintroducing FODMAPs

IBS can express itself in a variety of ways, and even two people with the same type of IBS may experience different symptoms and may respond differently to the same treatments. In addition, IBS symptoms may change over time.

The researchers at Monash University in Australia and dietitians who specialize in low-FODMAP diets recommend that a very strict low-FODMAP diet is adhered to initially for just a short period of time—two to eight weeks. Doing so will help mitigate IBS symptoms, identify trigger foods, and determine how well the diet is working for you. During this period it's important to avoid all foods that are moderate or high in FODMAPs. The key to success is diligence and commitment (and as a vegan, you're already in good supply of both of these).

This two-month trial should be followed by a period of food challenges, during which higher-FODMAP foods are reintroduced. This enables people with IBS to assess their tolerance to various FODMAP groups and ideally attain more variety in their diets. If your symptoms improve after the initial two-month period, you can gradually try reintroducing one higher-FODMAP food at a time to see how well you tolerate it. Start slowly, adding just a small portion of the food at one meal only and then waiting three to four days before trying it again or trying another higher-FODMAP food. Small amounts of higher-FODMAP foods may be better tolerated if all other foods at the meal are low in FODMAPs.

If you find that any quantity of higher-FODMAP foods induces symptoms, avoid those foods entirely and resume eating only FODMAP-safe choices. To help you stick with the diet and ensure a healthy balance, make sure you have plenty of variety: rotate the fruits, vegetables, and grains you eat each day to keep meals both interesting and nutritionally sound. Remember, your diet only needs to be as strict as your symptoms dictate!

For supersensitive people, however, reintroducing higher-FODMAP foods can be very difficult because symptoms may return even if very small quantities of these foods are consumed. These individuals may need to observe a strict low-FODMAP diet for a longer period to maintain symptom control. However, it's advised that you repeat unsuccessful food challenges occasionally because your symptoms and sensitivity to various foods will transform over time. In addition, reintroducing higher-FODMAP foods very gradually and in very small amounts can improve your tolerance to them.

Because adverse changes to the gut microbiome are associated with long-term adherence to a low-FODMAP diet, staying on a very restricted, very low-FODMAP diet permanently isn't recommended. It's important to find a balance between a low-FODMAP regimen and the occasional inclusion of moderate- to high-FODMAP foods while maintaining adequate symptom management. If you find that reintroducing higher-FODMAP foods is extremely challenging, you might want to consult with a dietitian familiar with both low-FODMAP and vegan diets. Knowledgeable dietitians can help in a variety of ways:

- They can identify food triggers other than FODMAPs.
- They can ensure that your diet is nutritionally adequate if you need to remain on a strict low-FODMAP diet for a longer period of time.
- They can suggest additional strategies to improve food tolerance.
- They can work with your health care provider to develop the best treatment plan for your needs.

The rechallenge phase will vary from person to person. Some people may be able to reintroduce a wide range of high-FODMAP foods and consume them regularly, while others may only be able to reintroduce a few specific foods very gradually or intermittently and consume them in only small amounts. Pick a smart time for the reintroduction phase, as trying to add higher-FODMAP foods while you're in the midst of a flare-up or during holidays or special occasions, for example, isn't a good idea. You might also find that some days or weeks you can tolerate higher-FODMAP foods better than other days or weeks, so allow yourself that flexibility and don't get discouraged if you need to occasionally or even frequently return to a stricter low-FODMAP plan until you feel better.

The low-FODMAP diet excludes all types of FODMAPs, even though not everyone with IBS will be intolerant to all of them. The purpose of the reintroduction phase is to determine which specific high-FODMAP foods you're most sensitive to. By systematically reintroducing individual foods, you will have an opportunity to identify your specific symptom triggers and potentially follow a less-restrictive diet.

Because everyone (and everyone's digestive system) is unique, you will need to formulate your own plan to reintroduce some higher-FODMAP items to discover your tolerance levels. A good place to start is by adding back small amounts of higher-FODMAP canned legumes—such as black beans, red beans, white beans, or peas—to your diet. Use quantities small enough to not cause significant symptoms but that are sufficient enough to gradually build up your prebiotic intake and encourage friendly bacterial growth in your gut. Alternatively, add back one of your favorite high-FODMAP foods—perhaps apple, avocado, cashews, dates, or mango—and try eating just a small amount of it.

Even after you complete the reintroduction phase, you probably won't end up eating the same diet that you did before you restricted your FODMAP intake. You will likely create your own modified version of the low-FODMAP vegan diet that includes some higher-FODMAP foods in quantities you can tolerate, while continuing to limit other foods in order to maintain good control of your symptoms. Bear in mind that IBS symptoms commonly vary over time, so even if you're not able to reintroduce many foods during your initial rechallenge, you may find that as your symptoms improve, you might be able to tolerate more higher-FODMAP options.

Maintaining Intestinal Fortitude

Although at first glance a low-FODMAP vegan diet may seem terribly restrictive, you'll be amazed by the wide variety of nutrient-dense foods from which you can choose. If you're concerned about getting adequate protein on a low-FODMAP vegan diet, know that there are quite a few protein-rich options available to you (see column B, table 11, opposite page). Below are just a few of the many recipes in this book that are packed with low-FODMAP plant-based protein:

Baked Zucchini and Potatoes with Greek Tofu Feta, *page 93*

Barbecued Tempeh Short Ribs, *page 88*

Breakfast Quinoa, *page 64*

Breakfast Scramble, *page 78*

Chickenless Chicken, *page 52*

Chickenless Chicken Salad, *page 52*

Chickenless Chicken Salad with Grapes and Pecans, *page 52*

Classic Lentil Loaf, *page 100*

Coconut-Curry Tofu and Veggie Stir-Fry, *page 81*

Creamy Lentil and Coconut Soup, *page 121*

Creamy Vegetable Soup, *page 120*

Eggplant, Spinach, and Lentil Bolognese with Pasta, *page 98*

Ginger-Glazed Tempeh Filets, *page 87*

Gingered Nut Butter Gravy, *page 109*

Greek Tofu Feta, *page 48*

Greek Tomato and Feta Salad, *page 48*

Green Bean and Walnut Pâté, *page 62*

Grilled Hummus Sandwich, *page 61*

Herbed Tempeh Nuggets, *page 51*

I Can't Believe It's Not Cheese Sauce, *page 60*

I Can't Believe It's Not Cheese Spread, *page 60*

I Can't Believe It's Not Grilled Cheese, *page 60*

Kale, Peanut, and Pineapple Stew, *page 96*

Lemon Rice with Kale, Mint, and Feta, *page 94*

Lemon-Pepper Tofu, *page 50*

Lentil and Walnut Pâté, *page 62*

Lentil Hummus, *page 61*

Lentil Salad with Chard and Tomatoes, *page 130*

Lentil Salad with Spinach and Tomatoes, *page 130*

Lentil-Chickpea Hummus, *page 61*

Maple-Miso Tofu, *page 50*

Minestrone, *page 124*

No-Bake Peanut Butter Granola Bars, *page 74*

Roasted Veggie and Legume Salad, *page 82*

Seasoned Pumpkin or Sunflower Seeds, *page 53*

Spicy Peanut Sauce, *page 110*

Tempeh Bacon, *page 49*

Teriyaki Tempeh, *page 90*

Toasted Pumpkin or Sunflower Seeds, *page 53*

Tofu, Chickpea, and Spinach Stir-Fry, *page 91*

Tofu Bacon Strips or Slabs, *page 49*

Two-Way Tempeh Salad, *page 127*

Walnut Pâté, *page 62*

Warm Nut Butter Gravy, *page 108*

Yum-Yum Sauce, *page 108*

Planning the Perfect Low-FODMAP Vegan Plate

On days when you're not up to thinking about food or cooking, you can easily fix a meal with little to no advance planning. Just check your fridge and pantry and then check table 11 (below). Choose low-FODMAP bread or a cooked starch from column A, a protein from column B, and one or more cooked or raw vegetables from column C, while keeping the selections from each column within the recommended portion sizes (see pages 19 to 24). Add your favorite low-FODMAP seasonings (see page 37 and pages 54 to 59) and/or the sauce or salad dressing of your choice (see pages 108 to 118), and your healthy, tummy-friendly plate will be ready to serve.

TABLE 11 PLANNING THE PERFECT LOW-FODMAP VEGAN PLATE

STARCH	PROTEIN	VEGETABLES	
CHOOSE 1	CHOOSE 1*	CHOOSE 1 OR MORE	
100% sourdough spelt or wheat bread	Chickpeas, canned	Alfalfa sprouts	Kale
Gluten-free pasta	Lentils, canned	Arugula, baby	Lettuce, all types
Gluten-free vegan bread	Low-FODMAP nut butter	Bamboo shoots	Mesclun
Millet, hulled	Low-FODMAP nuts	Bean sprouts	Olives
Polenta	Low-FODMAP seeds	Bell pepper	Parsnip
Potato	Peanut butter	Bok choy	Radicchio
Quinoa	Peanuts, unsalted roasted	Broccoli	Radishes
Rice, basmati	Seitan (check ingredients)	Cabbage, common green or red	Rutabaga
Rice, brown	Tahini	Carrot	Scallion greens
Rice, white	Tempeh, plain	Celeriac	Spinach, baby
Squash, kabocha	Tofu, superfirm or extra-firm	Chard/Swiss chard	Squash, patty pan
Sweet potato (very small or one-half medium)		Collard greens	Squash, spaghetti
Wild rice		Cucumber	Squash, yellow
Yam		Eggplant	Tomato, cherry or grape
		Endive	Tomato, globe
	*Also refer to the list on page 40 for specific high-protein recipes found in this book.	Fennel	Turnip
		Green beans	Water chestnuts
			Zucchini

Meal by Meal

When you don't feel up to snuff, having a list of menu ideas for every meal of the day or week can be helpful. This way, you don't need to give too much thought to figuring out what to eat or purchase. Table 12 provides some suggestions that you can follow to the letter or mix and match to your heart's content. If you need to eat smaller amounts of food at a time, use the menu suggestions as a general guide but divide up the options to create mini meals or snacks. You can then enjoy them throughout the day rather than eating everything on the menu at a single sitting.

Let's Get Cooking

All the recipes in this book were designed to be uncomplicated and extremely easy to prepare, regardless of your culinary expertise. They call for just a small number of ingredients, most of which are minimally processed, inexpensive, and readily available at well-stocked mainstream supermarkets and natural food stores. These are comforting, foundational recipes you can turn to day after day, whether you're feeling great or are tackling a flare-up. Plus, they've been tested many times over, so you can rest assured they're reliable and will work. And every one is bursting with spectacular flavor, not FODMAPs. Of course, each person's tastes and sensitivities are unique, so feel free to adjust the recipes and seasonings to your individual preferences and needs, as they were designed to be very adaptable.

You'll find recipes for low-FODMAP vegan staples, seasonings, and condiments, such as all-purpose herb blend, cheese spread, curry paste, feta cheese, hummus, ketchup, pickles, salsa, sriracha sauce, and vegetable stock, that aren't available on grocery store shelves but rival the taste of their high-FODMAP counterparts. They make it easy for you to not only prepare dishes from this book but to also adapt recipes from other sources that might otherwise be off limits. In addition, you'll discover fresh go-to favorites for every meal of the day, along with effortless treats and wholesome snacks. The recipes range from light to hearty, savory to sweet, and sedate to spicy, as well as everything in between, so regardless of your predilections, I've got your back. Many of the recipes include a number of variations, so you can customize them to suit your needs or mood or transform them to create endless diversity. In addition, all the recipes are naturally gluten-free, but if you have celiac disease or are allergic to wheat, avoid using seitan when it's listed as an option, make sure you purchase only certified gluten-free ingredients, and check product labels carefully.

When you don't feel well, it can be tough to figure out which foods to eat and what will pamper, not inflame, your delicate digestion. The ideas found earlier in this chapter and the recipes that follow provide a GPS for what to select. We're in this together, so let's get cookin'. Meet me in the kitchen!

TABLE 12 MEAL BY MEAL, DAY BY DAY

	BREAKFAST	LUNCH	DINNER	
DAY 1	Breakfast Quinoa (page 64) 1 serving suitable fruit Tea/Coffee	Two-Way Tempeh Salad (page 127) Lettuce or sprouts Gluten-free vegan crackers, 100% sourdough spelt or wheat bread, or gluten-free vegan bread 1 serving suitable fruit or fruit salad	Kale, Peanut, and Pineapple Stew (page 96) served over cooked quinoa, rice, or millet Dark Chocolate Tapioca Pudding (page 68)	1
DAY 2	Creamy Oatmeal Bowls (page 65) with banana and chocolate chips Tea/Coffee	Triple-Play Veggie Sandwich (page 126) 1 serving suitable fruit	Garden Vegetable Soup (page 124) Loaded Baked Potatoes (page 101) Maple-Vanilla Soft Serve (page 72)	2
DAY 3	Peanut Butter–Banana Instant Breakfast Drink (page 73) Toasted 100% sourdough spelt or wheat bread or gluten-free vegan bread, with low-FODMAP vegan butter or jam Tea/Coffee	I Can't Believe It's Not Grilled Cheese (page 60) Carrot sticks 1 serving suitable fruit or fruit salad	Tortilla Pull-Aparts (page 84) 1 serving suitable fruit or fruit salad	3
DAY 4	Low-FODMAP cold cereal with Almond Milk (page 46) Blueberries, sliced strawberries, diced kiwifruit, or sliced banana Tea/Coffee	Chickenless Chicken Salad (page 52) on a bed of romaine lettuce Sliced tomatoes 1 serving suitable fruit or fruit salad	Bliss Bowls (page 104) 1 serving suitable fruit or fruit salad	4
DAY 5	Pumpkin Pie Mousse (page 70) or No-Bake Peanut Butter Granola Bars (page 74) 1 serving suitable fruit Tea/Coffee	Tossed salad with radishes, cucumbers, and shredded carrots, topped with Greek Tofu Feta (page 48) Greek Lemon Vinaigrette (page 116)	Coconut-Curry Tofu and Veggie Stir-Fry (page 81) served over cooked rice Peanut Butter–Fudge Soft Serve (page 72)	5
DAY 6	Maple–Peanut Butter Oatmeal (page 66) Tea/Coffee	Green Bean and Walnut Pâté (page 62) Gluten-free vegan crackers, 100% sourdough spelt or wheat bread, or gluten-free vegan bread Mesclun salad with Noochy Dressing (page 117)	Eggplant and Spinach Bolognese with Pasta (page 98) 1 serving suitable fruit or fruit salad	6
DAY 7	Breakfast Scramble (page 78) Gluten-free vegan crackers Tea/Coffee	Lentil Salad with Chard and Tomatoes (page 130) Gluten-free vegan crackers, 100% sourdough spelt or wheat bread, or gluten-free vegan bread	Creamy Vegetable Soup (page 120) Gluten-free vegan crackers, 100% sourdough spelt or wheat bread, or gluten-free vegan bread Strawberry–Poppy Seed Soft Serve (page 72)	7

TABLE 13 COOKING TIMES FOR LOW-FODMAP GRAINS

GRAIN (1 CUP)	WATER	COOKING TIME	YIELD
Cornmeal polenta (coarsely ground yellow corn grits)	4 cups	15 to 20 minutes	2½ cups
Millet polenta or millet mashed "potatoes"*	3 cups	35 minutes	4 cups
Millet pilaf†	2 cups	15 to 20 minutes	3½ cups
Quinoa	2 cups	25 minutes	4 cups
Rice, basmati or long-grain white	2 cups	15 to 20 minutes	3 cups
Rice, brown	2½ cups	40 to 50 minutes (depending on variety)	3 to 4 cups
Wild rice‡	3 cups	50 to 60 minutes	3½ cups

*Millet prepared with extra water and a long cooking time will create a mush that's comparable to cornmeal polenta or mashed potatoes and may be used in similar ways. Season it with salt, pepper, and low-FODMAP vegan butter or extra-virgin olive oil to taste, stirring vigorously until creamy.

†Millet will taste best if it is toasted before cooking. Put it in the saucepan (dry or with a small amount of oil or low-FODMAP vegan butter) and heat over medium-high heat, stirring frequently, until it turns a rich golden brown and the grains are lightly toasted and fragrant, 4 to 5 minutes. Be careful not to let the grains burn. Because the saucepan will be hot, the water will sputter when you pour it in, so stand back to avoid getting burned.

‡Wild rice is cooked when the kernels puff open and are butterflied. If they are done cooking before all the water is absorbed, drain the excess liquid and let the rice rest, covered, for 5 to 10 minutes.

Low-FODMAP Staples

Almond Milk

MAKES 1 QUART

Per cup:

13 calories

0 g protein

0 g fat (0 g sat)

1 g carbs

74 mg sodium

2 mg calcium

0 g fiber

Most commercial brands of almond milk contain thickeners and other ingredients that aren't particularly healthy. And homemade almond milk recipes generally call for a large quantity of almonds, resulting in a product that's too rich and too high in FODMAPs to be well tolerated by people with IBS. In addition, most recipes call for sweetening the milk with dates, which are also high in FODMAPs. This recipe uses a safe ratio of almonds to water and just a tiny amount of cane sugar, resulting in a luxuriously creamy, light, and refreshing milk that can be used for both sweet and savory applications. It's also perfect for drinking, using in smoothies, or pouring over low-FODMAP breakfast cereals. For a richer, creamier version, see the variation that follows.

¼ **cup raw almonds, soaked in water with ¼ teaspoon sea salt for 6 hours** (see tip)

3½ **cups water, plus more as needed**

1 **teaspoon unbleached cane sugar**

Drain the almonds in a colander, rinse well, and drain again. Transfer to a high-powered blender (such as a Vitamix or Blendtec). Add the water and sugar and process on high speed until the almonds are completely pulverized, 1½ to 2 minutes. Put a nut milk bag (see box, opposite page) over a large bowl or large measuring cup and pour the milk through it. Slowly and gently squeeze the bag (from the top downward) to release the milk. Continue to squeeze the bag until all the liquid has been extracted.

Pour the milk into a clean glass jar. Add more water as needed to make 4 cups of milk. Seal tightly and refrigerate. Stored in a sealed jar in the refrigerator, the milk will keep for about 5 days. Shake well before using.

TIP If you'd like to soak the almonds longer than 6 hours (which I recommend doing if you have the time), put them in the refrigerator. The longer they soak, the softer and easier to process they'll become. I like to keep almonds soaking in the fridge so I can make almond milk on a whim, without any advance prep.

NUTS ABOUT NUT MILK BAGS

A nut milk bag is essential for making the best almond milk. A poor-quality nut milk bag or alternatives such as cheesecloth won't provide good extraction of the almond pulp and will result in a thin, watery product. If that happens, you will need to use more almonds next time to achieve the same outcome that a smaller amount of almonds and a high-quality nut milk bag would produce.

The optimal and most durable nut milk bags are made of hemp and cotton (preferably organic). They're more expensive than nylon, but they'll last a very long time and will provide the finest filtration possible, making for a very smooth, delicious, and surprisingly white and rich-tasting almond milk with just a small quantity of nuts. After filtering the milk, discard the almond pulp, turn the nut milk bag inside out, and wash the bag by hand using a little dish detergent and white vinegar. This will keep the bag clean and fresh smelling. Rinse the bag thoroughly and let it air-dry completely before storing.

Chocolate Almond Milk Increase the sugar to ¼ cup. After straining the milk, return it to the blender and add 4 tablespoons of unsweetened cocoa powder. Process until well incorporated.

Rich Almond Milk Increase the amount of almonds to ½ cup. Use as is or with any of the other variations.

Strawberry Almond Milk Increase the sugar to ¼ cup. After straining the milk, return it to the blender and add 1½ cups of hulled whole strawberries (about 12 large). Process until smooth and well incorporated.

Vanilla Almond Milk Increase the sugar to 1 tablespoon and add ½ teaspoon of vanilla extract.

Greek Tofu Feta

MAKES 5 SERVINGS

Per serving:

108 calories

10 g protein

6 g fat (1 g sat)

3 g carbs

148 mg sodium

50 mg calcium

1 g fiber

Tart, tangy, salty vegan feta is easy to make, plus it's so versatile. Of course it's great mixed into salads, but you can also toss it with pasta dishes or pair it with cantaloupe and grapes. Crumble it to use as a sandwich filling, or sprinkle it over mashed potatoes or creamy polenta (see table 13, page 44). It's an essential element in Baked Zucchini and Potatoes with Greek Tofu Feta (page 93) and an outstanding addition to Bliss Bowls (page 104), Loaded Baked Potatoes (page 101), or Tortilla Pull-Aparts (page 84).

½ **cup water**

½ **cup cider vinegar**

¼ **cup freshly squeezed lemon juice**

2 **tablespoons chickpea or light miso**

1 **tablespoon dried oregano**

1 **tablespoon garlic-infused olive oil**

1 **teaspoon sea salt**

12 **ounces superfirm or extra-firm tofu, pressed** (see box, page 28) **and cubed** (see tip)

To make the brine, put the water, vinegar, lemon juice, miso, oregano, oil, and salt in a large bowl and whisk until well combined and the miso is fully incorporated. Add the tofu and gently toss, using your hands, until each piece is well coated with the brine. Take care not to break the cubes. Transfer the tofu and brine to a glass storage container, cover, and refrigerate for 24 to 48 hours before using. If all the cubes aren't submerged in the brine, gently tilt the container every few hours to ensure all pieces stay well coated. Store the feta in the brine in a sealed container in the refrigerator.

Greek Tomato and Feta Salad Seed 1 large, ripe tomato and cut it into bite-sized pieces. Transfer to a small bowl or serving dish. Add ¼ cup of drained Greek Tofu Feta, crumbled or in cubes, along with 6 Greek olives, a pinch of oregano, and a pinch of freshly ground black pepper. Drizzle with extra-virgin olive oil to taste. Makes 1 serving.

TIP If you only have access to tofu in 1-pound packages, you can use the entire package. There is no need to increase the amount of brine, but you will need to tilt the storage container regularly to ensure all pieces stay coated with the brine. Makes 6 servings.

Note: Analysis includes one-quarter of the brine ingredients, as the brine is not completely absorbed into the tofu.

Tofu Bacon Strips or Slabs

To keep the fat under control, this vegan bacon is baked rather than fried. Using well-pressed superfirm tofu, marinating it for several hours, and browning it thoroughly in the oven are the keys to achieving chewy, deeply flavored vegan bacon strips or slabs, perfect for a low-FODMAP BLT with vegan mayo.

8 ounces superfirm or extra-firm tofu, well pressed (see box, page 28)

3 tablespoons reduced-sodium tamari

2 tablespoons pure maple syrup

1 tablespoon nutritional yeast flakes (optional but highly recommended)

1 teaspoon extra-virgin olive oil or safflower oil

¼ teaspoon liquid smoke

MAKES 32 BACON STRIPS OR 8 SLABS, 4 SERVINGS

Per serving:

129 calories

9 g protein

5 g fat (1 g sat)

9 g carbs

554 mg sodium

115 mg calcium

1 g fiber

For strips, cut the tofu crosswise into 16 very thin slices, about 1 inch wide, 3½ inches long, and ⅛ inch thick. Then cut each slice in half lengthwise to make 32 strips, about ½ inch wide. Arrange the strips in a single layer in a 13 x 9-inch baking pan or on two large, flat plates.

For slabs, cut the tofu crosswise into 8 thin slices, about 1 inch wide, 3½ inches long, and ¼ inch thick. Arrange the slabs in a single layer in a 13 x 9-inch glass baking pan.

Put the tamari, maple syrup, optional nutritional yeast, oil, and liquid smoke in a measuring cup or small bowl and whisk until well combined. Spoon evenly over the tofu. Turn the strips or slabs over carefully so they don't break, dipping each one into the marinade that remains in the pan so that all the pieces are coated well on all sides. Cover tightly with plastic wrap and let marinate in the refrigerator for at least 1 hour or up to 24 hours, turning the strips or slabs over occasionally.

Preheat the oven to 400 degrees F. Line a baking sheet with parchment paper or a silicone baking mat. Arrange the tofu in a single layer on the lined baking sheet. Don't let the pieces touch or overlap or they won't cook properly. Bake for 12 minutes. Carefully turn the strips or slabs over and bake until deep golden brown, 10 to 12 minutes longer. Keep a close eye on the strips, especially during the last few minutes of baking, to ensure they don't burn (see tip). Serve warm or cover tightly and chill thoroughly before serving. Store in a sealed container in the refrigerator.

Tempeh Bacon Replace the tofu with 8 ounces of tempeh, cut crosswise into four equal pieces. Put the tempeh in a medium saucepan, cover with water, and bring to a gentle simmer over medium-high heat. Decrease the heat to medium-low and simmer gently for 10 minutes. Drain well and pat dry. Let cool, then slice each piece very thinly crosswise into 8 strips, about 3½ inches long, for a total of 32 strips. Marinate and bake as directed.

TIP Strive to make the strips or slabs equal in thickness. Thinner pieces will cook faster, and thicker ones may need to bake a little longer. But if they're all the same thickness, they should be done at the same time.

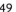

Maple-Miso Tofu

MAKES 5 SERVINGS

Per serving:

178 calories

13 g protein

8 g fat (1 g sat)

14 g carbs

521 mg sodium

168 mg calcium

2 g fiber

Using a modicum of staple ingredients, you can create chewy, flavor-infused tofu with very little effort or cleanup. Glazed with a mix of miso, tamari, and maple syrup, these tasty morsels make a great addition to Bliss Bowls (page 104), pasta, or salads, and the slices make an excellent base for Tortilla Pull-Aparts (page 84) or low-FODMAP sandwiches.

3 tablespoons pure maple syrup

2 tablespoons chickpea or light miso

2 tablespoons reduced-sodium tamari

1 tablespoon garlic-infused olive oil

1 pound superfirm or extra-firm tofu, pressed (see box, page 28) **and cut into ½-inch cubes or slices**

Preheat the oven to 350 degrees F. Line a large roasting pan with parchment paper or a silicone baking mat.

    Put the maple syrup, miso, tamari, and oil in a large bowl and whisk vigorously until smooth and well combined. Add the tofu and gently toss, using your hands, until each piece is well coated with the miso mixture. Take care to not break the pieces. Transfer the tofu and any sauce remaining in the bowl to the lined roasting pan and carefully arrange it in a single layer. Bake for 30 minutes, until golden brown. Serve warm or cover tightly and chill thoroughly before serving. Store in a sealed container in the refrigerator.

Lemon-Pepper Tofu

MAKES 5 SERVINGS

Per serving:

138 calories

12 g protein

8 g fat (1 g sat)

5 g carbs

175 mg sodium

165 mg calcium

2 g fiber

Enjoy this tart and spicy tofu in a sandwich, using low-FODMAP bread, or a wrap, using brown rice tortillas, along with lettuce, tomato, cucumber, and vegan mayo. Alternatively, use it as the base for Tortilla Pull-Aparts (page 84), or slice or dice it and add it to Bliss Bowls (page 104), gluten-free pasta with Good-to-Your-Gut Marinara Sauce (page 118), Ten-Minute One-Pan Pasta (page 97), stir-fried veggies, or salads.

1 pound superfirm or extra-firm tofu, pressed (see box, page 28)

5 tablespoons freshly squeezed lemon juice

1 tablespoon extra-virgin olive oil or garlic-infused olive oil

1 tablespoon reduced-sodium tamari

1½ teaspoons freshly ground black pepper

1 teaspoon dried thyme, well crushed between your fingers

1 teaspoon grated lemon zest (optional)

1 teaspoon balsamic vinegar

Cut the tofu into ¼- to ½-inch-thick slices. Oil a large roasting pan (preferably nonstick).

Arrange the tofu in a single layer in the prepared pan. Don't let the slices touch or overlap or they won't cook properly. Put the lemon juice, oil, tamari, pepper, thyme, optional lemon zest, and vinegar in a small jar, seal tightly, and shake until well combined. Pour evenly over the tofu. Let marinate for 30 minutes, shaking or tilting the pan occasionally to ensure all pieces are well coated with the marinade.

Preheat the oven to 350 degrees F. Bake for 30 minutes. Serve warm or cover tightly and chill thoroughly before serving. Store in a sealed container in the refrigerator.

Herbed Tempeh Nuggets

These tender, flavor-packed nuggets are fabulous tossed with salads, pasta, rice, or stir-fries . . . or just eaten out of hand as a snack.

8 ounces tempeh, cut into ½-inch cubes

2½ tablespoons balsamic vinegar

2½ tablespoons reduced-sodium tamari

1 tablespoon All-Purpose Herb Blend
(page 55)

1 tablespoon garlic-infused olive oil

¼ teaspoon crushed red pepper flakes

¼ teaspoon freshly ground black pepper

Pinch sea salt

1 tablespoon safflower or coconut oil

MAKES 4 SERVINGS

Per serving:
186 calories
12 g protein
13 g fat (2 g sat)
7 g carbs
476 mg sodium
64 mg calcium
0 g fiber

Put the tempeh in a medium saucepan. Cover with water and bring to a gentle simmer over medium-high heat. Decrease the heat to medium-low and simmer gently for 10 minutes. Drain well and pat dry. Transfer the tempeh to a medium bowl.

Put the vinegar, tamari, herb blend, garlic-infused oil, red pepper flakes, pepper, and salt in a small bowl and whisk to combine. Pour over the tempeh and toss gently until evenly coated. Cover and let marinate in the refrigerator for 1 to 24 hours.

To cook, heat the safflower oil in a large skillet (preferably nonstick) over medium heat. Add the tempeh and any remaining liquid and seasonings in the bowl and cook, stirring and turning the tempeh frequently, until well browned on all sides, 10 to 12 minutes. Serve warm or cover tightly and chill thoroughly before serving. Store in a sealed container in the refrigerator.

Chickenless Chicken

MAKES 5 SERVINGS

Per serving:

119 calories

13 g protein

5 g fat (1 g sat)

4 g carbs

600 mg sodium

176 mg calcium

2 g fiber

This minimalist recipe is a reliable staple because it's so simple and remarkably adaptable. You can slice it and add it to Bliss Bowls (page 104) or Tortilla Pull-Aparts (page 84), dice it to use in Chickenless Chicken Salad (see variation), or cube it and add it to Ten-Minute One-Pan Pasta (page 97) or a fresh green salad.

1 pound superfirm or extra-firm tofu, pressed (see box, page 28)

¾ cup water or Good-to-Your-Gut Vegetable Stock (page 58)

¼ cup reduced-sodium tamari

2 teaspoons nutritional yeast flakes (optional)

Cut the tofu crosswise into 15 thin slabs, about 1 inch wide, 3½ inches long, and ¼ inch thick. Arrange in a single layer in a large roasting pan or two 13 x 9-inch baking pans. Don't overlap the slices. Combine the water and tamari in a small measuring cup or bowl. Whisk in the optional nutritional yeast and pour over the tofu. Let marinate for 30 minutes, turning once or twice if the slices aren't fully submerged.

Preheat the oven to 400 degrees F. Line a baking sheet with parchment paper or a silicone baking mat. Remove the tofu from the marinade and discard the marinade. Arrange the tofu in a single layer on the lined baking sheet. Don't let the slices touch or overlap or they won't cook properly. Bake for 10 to 12 minutes. Carefully turn the slices over and bake for 10 to 12 minutes longer, until deep golden brown. Serve warm or cover tightly and chill thoroughly before serving. Store in a sealed container in the refrigerator.

Chickenless Chicken Salad Slice 1 pound of baked Chickenless Chicken into very thin strips. Transfer to a medium bowl. Add ½ cup of diced bell pepper (any color), ¼ cup of diced celery, and ¼ cup of thinly sliced scallion greens. Put ¾ cup of vegan mayonnaise and 2 teaspoons of Dijon, spicy brown, or yellow mustard in a small bowl and stir until well combined. Add to the chicken mixture and toss gently until all the ingredients are evenly distributed.

Chickenless Chicken Salad with Grapes and Pecans Dice 1 pound of baked Chickenless Chicken. Transfer to a medium bowl. Add 1 cup of vegan mayonnaise, 1 cup of seedless red grapes, halved lengthwise, ½ cup chopped toasted pecans (see variation, page 53), 5 tablespoons of sweetened dried cranberries, ½ teaspoon sea salt, and ½ teaspoon freshly ground black pepper. Toss gently until all the ingredients are evenly distributed.

Toasted Pumpkin or Sunflower Seeds

Pumpkin and sunflower seeds add extra flavor, protein, and crunch when sprinkled over salads, Bliss Bowls (page 104), Loaded Baked Potatoes (page 101), steamed vegetables, or whole grains. They're also great for a quick snack on the go, especially when well seasoned (see variation), but limit the portion size to one to two tablespoons of pumpkin seeds or two teaspoons of sunflower seeds to stay within low-FODMAP guidelines.

½ cup raw pumpkin seeds or sunflower seeds
2 teaspoons reduced-sodium tamari (optional)

Preheat the oven to 375 degrees F. Line a baking sheet with parchment paper or a silicone baking mat. Put the seeds and optional tamari in a small bowl and stir until evenly coated. Spread in a single layer on the lined baking sheet. Bake for 8 to 12 minutes, until the seeds are lightly toasted and fragrant. Immediately transfer to a plate to cool. Break up any clumps with your hands. (The tamari can cause the seeds to stick together.) Cool completely before storing. Store in a tightly sealed container at room temperature.

Seasoned Pumpkin or Sunflower Seeds Add 1 teaspoon of Tan-Tan Spice Mix or Sweet-n-Savory Spice Mix (page 55) and a pinch of cayenne along with the tamari. (Warning: These are addictively delicious.)

Toasted Nuts Replace the seeds with ½ cup of pecans, walnuts, macadamia nuts, or whole or slivered almonds.

TIP If you use toasted seeds frequently, make a double batch. The toasted seeds store well, and the baking time will be the same.

MAKES ½ CUP

Per 2 tablespoons (pumpkin seeds):
85 calories
5 g protein
8 g fat (1 g sat)
2 g carbs
0 mg sodium
10 mg calcium
1 g fiber

Per 1 tablespoon (sunflower seeds):
50 calories
2 g protein
4 g fat (1 g sat)
2 g carbs
0 mg sodium
10 mg calcium
1 g fiber

Mild Hot Chile Paste

MAKES 1 CUP

Per tablespoon:
25 calories
1 g protein
0 g fat (0 g sat)
5 g carbs
249 mg sodium
6 mg calcium
1 g fiber

This salty, spicy paste is mild compared to most hot chile pastes. Thinned with a little water, it's remarkably similar to Korean gochujang, an essential seasoning sauce in Korean cuisine. Additional water will turn it into a flavorful liquid that can replace Tabasco or other commercial hot sauces. A dab of the paste mixed into foods will pump up the flavor considerably. Stir a spoonful into rice or other gluten-free grains, stir-fries, marinades, sauces, or vegan mayonnaise. It can also be used to make a delectable low-FODMAP Thai curry paste (see the variation that follows).

4 tablespoons paprika

3 tablespoons unbleached cane sugar

½ teaspoon cayenne

5 tablespoons chickpea or light miso

2 tablespoons reduced-sodium tamari

3 tablespoons water

Put the paprika, sugar, and cayenne in a small saucepan (preferably nonstick) and whisk or stir to combine. Add the miso and tamari and stir until smooth and well blended. Add the water, 1 tablespoon at a time, until smooth and well incorporated. Heat over medium-low heat, stirring almost constantly, just until the sugar is melted, 2 to 3 minutes. Transfer to a glass storage container and let cool. Stored in a covered container in the refrigerator, the paste will keep for 6 months.

Mild Hot Sauce Put a small amount of the warm or chilled paste in a small bowl. Gradually whisk in a small amount of water, 1 teaspoon at a time, to create a smooth, thick sauce, using just enough water to achieve the desired consistency. Use immediately or cover tightly and store in the refrigerator.

Thai Red Curry Paste Put 2 tablespoons of the warm or chilled paste in a small bowl. Whisk in 2 teaspoons of freshly squeezed lemon juice, 2 teaspoons of garlic-infused olive oil, 1 teaspoon of ground coriander, 1 teaspoon of peeled and grated fresh ginger, ½ teaspoon of ground cumin, and ¼ teaspoon of ground turmeric. Cover tightly and store in the refrigerator. Use in any recipe that calls for Thai red or green curry paste.

All-Purpose Herb Blend

Use this tasty, salt-free, FODMAP-free, all-purpose herbal mix to heighten the flavor of soups, salads, dressings, grains, gravies, sauces, and vegetables.

MAKES ½ CUP

2 tablespoons dried thyme, well crushed between your fingers

2 tablespoons dried oregano

4 teaspoons rubbed sage

2 teaspoons dried basil

2 teaspoons dried marjoram

2 teaspoons dried parsley

2 teaspoons dried rosemary, well crushed between your fingers

Put all the ingredients in a small jar, seal tightly, and shake well to combine.

Tan-Tan Spice Mix

This aromatic, full-flavored mixture was inspired by an intriguing spice combination of the same name that's common to North African cuisine. The bold blend of sweet, hot, and savory tastes will instantly ramp up the flavor of any soup or stew. It's a terrific all-purpose seasoning and is particularly splendid when sprinkled over hot rice or vegetables.

MAKES ½ CUP

5 tablespoons paprika

2 teaspoons dried basil, crushed between your fingers

1 teaspoon ground ginger

½ teaspoon freshly ground black pepper

½ teaspoon ground allspice

½ teaspoon ground cardamom

½ teaspoon ground cinnamon

½ teaspoon ground cumin

½ teaspoon ground fenugreek

½ teaspoon ground nutmeg

½ teaspoon ground turmeric

¼ teaspoon ground cloves

Put all the ingredients in a small jar, seal tightly, and shake well to combine.

Sweet-n-Savory Spice Mix

This fragrant blend combines both sweet and savory Indian spices. It adds a vibrant flavor to tomato, potato, and grain dishes and is especially delicious as a soup or vegetable seasoning. On toasted seeds (see Seasoned Pumpkin or Sunflower Seeds, page 53) it's irresistible.

MAKES ½ CUP

2 tablespoons ground coriander

2 tablespoons ground cumin

2 tablespoons paprika

1 tablespoon ground fenugreek

2 teaspoons ground cardamom

2 teaspoons ground cinnamon

2 teaspoons ground cloves

2 teaspoons ground nutmeg

½ teaspoon sea salt

½ teaspoon freshly ground black pepper

½ teaspoon ground turmeric

Put all the ingredients in a small jar, seal tightly, and shake well to combine.

Good-to-Your-Gut Sriracha Sauce

MAKES 1½ CUPS

Per tablespoon:

17 calories

0 g protein

1 g fat (0.1 g sat)

3 g carbs

259 mg sodium

1 mg calcium

0 g fiber

Although authentic sriracha sauce, also known as rooster sauce, is quite heavy on garlic and heat, this FODMAP-friendly version is a close facsimile and mighty tasty. If you use jarred roasted red peppers, it can be whipped up in mere minutes. It's a great sauce to spoon over any gluten-free grain; makes an excellent condiment for tofu, tempeh, or stir-fries; and adds a fiery kick to mashed potatoes or polenta. Just keep in mind the heat level; you'll want to use it in small amounts if you're sensitive to spicy seasonings.

2 cups roasted red bell peppers (about 4 peppers), **rinsed well and drained** (see recipe, opposite page)

¼ cup rice vinegar

2 tablespoons light brown sugar

1 tablespoon garlic-infused olive oil

1 tablespoon Tabasco or Mild Hot Sauce (page 54)

1½ teaspoons sea salt

¼ teaspoon cayenne

Remove and discard any blackened skin from the peppers. Split open the peppers and remove and discard any seeds clinging to the interior or ribs. Put the peppers, vinegar, brown sugar, oil, Tabasco, salt, and cayenne in a food processor or blender and pulse or process on low speed until combined but not quite smooth. The mixture should have some texture, but if you prefer a smooth sauce, pulse or process a little longer. Pour into a deep, medium saucepan (preferably nonstick) and bring to a simmer over medium heat. Decrease the heat to medium-low, partially cover to minimize splatters, and simmer, stirring almost constantly, until slightly thickened, about 20 minutes. Remove from the heat and let cool. Stored in a covered container in the refrigerator, the sauce will keep for about 2 weeks.

Sriracha Dressing Put 3 tablespoons of vegan mayonnaise, 1 tablespoon of Good-to-Your-Gut Sriracha Sauce, 1 teaspoon of freshly squeezed lime juice, and ¼ teaspoon of reduced-sodium tamari in a small bowl or measuring cup and stir or whisk until smooth and well combined. Makes ¼ cup.

Sriracha Mayo Put 3 tablespoons of vegan mayonnaise and 1 tablespoon of Good-to-Your-Gut Sriracha Sauce in a small bowl or measuring cup and stir or whisk until smooth and well combined. Makes ¼ cup.

Sriracha-Mustard Mayo Put 4 tablespoons of vegan mayonnaise, 1 tablespoon of Good-to-Your-Gut Sriracha Sauce, and 1 tablespoon of yellow mustard in a small bowl or measuring cup and stir or whisk until smooth and well combined. Makes 6 tablespoons.

Roasted Red Peppers

If you don't have access to jarred roasted peppers, it's easy to roast your own at home.

6 large red bell peppers

1½ tablespoons extra-virgin olive oil (optional)

Preheat the oven to 450 degrees F. Line a rimmed baking sheet with parchment paper or a silicone baking mat.

Put the peppers on the lined baking sheet and roast, turning the peppers as each side browns, until they have darkened and collapsed, 50 to 60 minutes.

Transfer to a large bowl and cover with a plate or foil. Let the peppers steam until cool enough to handle. Remove and discard the stems, skins, and seeds using your fingers. Don't worry if the peppers fall apart. Transfer to a storage container, drizzle with the optional oil (the oil will help the peppers keep longer), and toss gently until evenly coated. Cover tightly and store in the refrigerator.

MAKES 6 PEPPERS

Per pepper:
31 calories
1 g protein
0 g fat (0 g sat)
6 g carbs
4 mg sodium
1 mg calcium
2 g fiber

Good-to-Your-Gut Ketchup

One of the biggest challenges of a low-FODMAP diet is finding safe condiments. Ketchup is among them, as virtually all commercial ketchups contain onion. This kind-to-your-tummy version is as tasty as it is simple to make.

1½ cups no-salt-added tomato purée

¼ cup white wine vinegar or cider vinegar

2 tablespoons unbleached cane sugar

2 tablespoons light brown sugar

½ teaspoon dry mustard

½ teaspoon sea salt

¼ teaspoon ground cinnamon

¼ teaspoon ground coriander

⅛ teaspoon freshly ground black pepper

⅛ teaspoon ground cloves

Put all the ingredients in a deep, medium saucepan (preferably nonstick) and bring to a simmer over medium heat. Decrease the heat to medium-low, partially cover to minimize splatters, and simmer, stirring occasionally, until reduced and thickened, about 40 minutes. Adjust the heat as necessary to maintain a simmer, and stir more frequently toward the end when the ketchup has begun to thicken. Stand back when lifting the lid and stirring to avoid getting splattered or burned. Let cool completely before storing. Stored in a covered container in the refrigerator, the ketchup will keep for 3 weeks.

MAKES 1¼ CUPS

Per 1 tablespoon:
16 calories
0 g protein
0 g fat (0 g sat)
4 g carbs
50 mg sodium
0 mg calcium
0 g fiber

Good-to-Your-Gut Vegetable Stock

MAKES 10 CUPS

Packaged vegetable broth and bouillon cubes invariably contain onion. Fortunately, it's not difficult or time-consuming to make a rich vegetable stock at home that's low in FODMAPs and kind to your belly. This stock is flavorful and soothing—ideal to use as a base for soups or sauces or just to sip from a mug when you need something light and comforting.

1 tablespoon garlic-infused olive oil

2 large carrots, scrubbed and sliced into 1-inch pieces

2 large Swiss chard leaves (any variety), with stems, coarsely sliced, or 1 zucchini or summer squash, sliced into 1-inch pieces

1 bell pepper (any color), sliced into 1-inch pieces

1 large tomato, quartered

12 scallions, green part only, coarsely chopped

8 sprigs fresh parsley

1 large sprig fresh thyme

1 large sprig fresh rosemary

2 bay leaves

6 whole black peppercorns

3 cloves (optional)

12 cups water

Put the oil in a large soup pot and heat over medium-high heat. When hot, add the carrots, chard, bell pepper, tomato, and scallions. Cook, stirring frequently, for 10 minutes. Add the parsley, thyme, rosemary, bay leaves, peppercorns, optional cloves, and water and bring to a boil. Decrease the heat to medium and simmer, uncovered, stirring occasionally, for 45 minutes. Strain through a fine-mesh strainer and discard the solids. Let cool, then store in a sealed container in the refrigerator. Alternatively, pour into small containers or ice-cube trays (for ease of use) and store in the freezer.

TIP This recipe is a great way to use up any vegetables and vegetable scraps that you have on hand, such as celery root (celeriac), eggplant (flesh and/or peels), fresh or dried herbs (marjoram, oregano, parsley, sage), green beans, kale (leaves and/or stems), or potato peels. Store them in a sealed container in the refrigerator as they accumulate and then just toss them in with the carrots at the start of the recipe. If you increase the quantity of vegetables substantially, use an additional tablespoon of garlic-infused olive oil and add an additional cup or two of water.

Zucchini in a Pickle

Perfect for adding a gratifying crunch to low-FODMAP sandwiches, these crisp slices are pickled overnight in the refrigerator—no canning required! They're pleasingly tart with just a hint of sweetness. To put other vegetables in a pickle, see the variations that follow.

1 cup cider vinegar

6 tablespoons unbleached cane sugar

1½ tablespoons kosher salt, pickling salt, or white sea salt

1 cup cold water

1 sprig fresh dill, or ½ teaspoon dried dill weed (optional)

½ teaspoon brown or yellow mustard seeds (optional)

½ teaspoon whole black, white, or mixed peppercorns (optional)

1 pound young or small zucchini, cut into ¼-inch-thick slices

MAKES 1 QUART

Per 6 slices, about ½ cup:

19 calories

1 g protein

0 g fat (0 g sat)

4 g carbs

339 mg sodium

10 mg calcium

1 g fiber

To make the brine, put the vinegar, sugar, and salt in a small saucepan and bring to a boil over high heat. Remove from the heat and whisk until the sugar and salt are dissolved. Whisk in the cold water.

Put the optional dill, optional mustard seeds, and optional peppercorns in a clean, widemouthed, 1-quart jar. Pack the zucchini tightly into the jar. Pour in the brine, leaving about one-half inch of headroom. Press the zucchini down gently so all the slices are submerged. Let cool completely, about 1 hour. Tap the jar gently on the countertop to remove any air bubbles. Seal the jar tightly and turn it gently to distribute the seasonings evenly. Refrigerate for 24 hours before serving. Stored in the sealed jar in the refrigerator, the pickles will keep for at least 1 month.

Carrots in a Pickle Replace the zucchini with 1 pound of young spring carrots, trimmed, peeled, and halved lengthwise, or 1 pound of bagged baby carrots, halved lengthwise.

Cucumbers in a Pickle Replace the zucchini with 1 pound of Kirby cucumbers, cut lengthwise into quarters (to make spears) or sliced into ¼-inch-thick rounds.

Green Beans in a Pickle Replace the zucchini with 12 ounces of trimmed green beans or haricot verts.

Mixed Veggies in a Pickle Use any combination of carrots, cucumbers, green beans, bell pepper strips, radishes, and zucchini.

Pickle Relish Finely chop any amount of drained pickles. If desired, mix in a small amount of finely chopped pimientos for added color and flavor.

TIP The brine can be used for a second batch of pickles. Just prepare the zucchini or other vegetables (see variations), add them to the brine, and let pickle in the refrigerator for 48 hours. They will take longer to pickle because the brine will be cold. After the second batch is consumed, start a new batch with fresh brine.

Note: Analysis includes one-quarter of the brine ingredients, as the brine is not completely absorbed into the zucchini.

I Can't Believe It's Not Cheese Spread

MAKES 1⅓ CUPS, 5 SERVINGS

Per serving:

183 calories

6 g protein

13 g fat (2 g sat)

11 g carbs

246 mg sodium

20 mg calcium

3 g fiber

Most vegan cheeses contain high-FODMAP ingredients, such as cashews and onion or garlic powder. This deceptively simple cheese spread offers plenty of cheesy flavor without dairy products, while keeping the protein high and the FODMAPs low. It's fabulous as a sandwich filling, a base for Tortilla Pull-Aparts (page 84), or a topping for Loaded Baked Potatoes (page 101). Or you can just lick it off a spoon.

½ cup no-salt-added canned chickpeas, rinsed well and drained

¼ cup water

3 tablespoons tahini

3 tablespoons no-salt-added creamy peanut butter

2 tablespoons nutritional yeast flakes

2 tablespoons chickpea or light miso

2 tablespoons freshly squeezed lemon juice

1 tablespoon garlic-infused olive oil

Pinch smoked paprika (optional)

Pinch sea salt (optional)

Put all the ingredients in a food processor or high-powered blender and process until smooth, 2 to 3 minutes. Transfer to a sealed container and refrigerate for 24 hours before serving to let the flavors meld. Store in a sealed container in the refrigerator.

Chive Cheese Spread Pulse or stir 2 tablespoons of dried chives into the spread after processing.

I Can't Believe It's Not Cheese Sauce Increase the water to ½ cup. Add more water as needed, 1 teaspoon at a time, to achieve the desired consistency. To heat the sauce, put the desired amount in a saucepan and warm over low heat; do not boil.

I Can't Believe It's Not Grilled Cheese Spread 2 tablespoons of the cheese spread on a slice of 100% sourdough spelt or wheat bread or gluten-free vegan bread. Top with 3 slices of seeded tomato. Cover with another slice of bread. Brown both sides of the sandwich in melted low-FODMAP vegan butter in a skillet.

Orange Cheese Sauce Add ¼ cup of additional water and ¼ cup of roasted red bell pepper. Process until no flecks of the bell pepper remain. Add more water as needed, 1 teaspoon at a time, to achieve the desired consistency. To heat the sauce, put the desired amount in a saucepan and warm over low heat; do not boil.

Orange Cheese Spread Replace the water with ¼ cup of roasted red bell pepper (see box, page 57). Process until no flecks of the bell pepper remain.

Lentil Hummus

Hummus is a vegan staple, but it's traditionally made with chickpeas, which keeps the acceptable portion size on a low-FODMAP diet quite small. In addition, hummus is typically loaded with garlic and tahini, which pushes it way out of the safe zone for people with IBS. This hummus is made with canned lentils instead of chickpeas, includes garlic-infused oil instead of garlic, and contains just a smidge of tahini, making it possible to have larger portions, because who wants to stop at just a nibble?

MAKES 1 CUP, 4 SERVINGS

Per serving:
203 calories
10 g protein
10 g fat (1 g sat)
16 g carbs
123 mg sodium
33 mg calcium
8 g fiber

1 can (15 ounces) **no-salt-added lentils, rinsed well and drained**

2 tablespoons tahini

2 tablespoons no-salt-added creamy peanut butter or additional tahini

2 tablespoons freshly squeezed lemon juice

1 teaspoon garlic-infused olive oil

¼ teaspoon ground coriander

¼ teaspoon ground cumin

¼ teaspoon ground turmeric

¼ teaspoon sea salt

¼ teaspoon freshly ground black pepper

Pinch smoked paprika (optional)

Pinch cayenne (optional)

Paprika, for garnish

Put all the ingredients in a food processor or high-speed blender and process until smooth, stopping once or twice as needed to scrape down the container. Store in a sealed container in the refrigerator. Garnish with paprika just before serving.

Grilled Hummus Sandwich Spread 2 tablespoons of Lentil-Hummus or Lentil-Chickpea Hummus (see below) on a slice of 100% sourdough spelt or wheat bread or gluten-free vegan bread. Top with 3 slices of seeded tomato. Cover with another slice of bread. Brown both sides of the sandwich in melted low-FODMAP vegan butter in a skillet.

Lentil-Chickpea Hummus Use 1 cup of canned lentils and ¾ cup of canned chickpeas, rinsed well and drained. Proceed with the recipe as directed.

Zucchini Hummus Replace the lentils with 1⅔ cups of diced or finely chopped raw zucchini and add 1 tablespoon of additional tahini or peanut butter. Proceed with the recipe as directed. Stir well before serving.

Walnut Pâté

MAKES ¾ CUP, 4 SERVINGS

Per serving:

214 calories

5 g protein

21 g fat (2 g sat)

5 g carbs

177 mg sodium

5 mg calcium

2 g fiber

This exquisite pâté is rich and elegant enough to serve at a party, but don't hold it in reserve just for guests. It makes a delectable spread for sandwiches or crackers, a tasty base for Tortilla Pull-Aparts (page 84), and a great topping for baked potatoes too (see page 101). Be sure to also try all the variations that follow.

1 cup raw walnuts, soaked in water and a pinch of sea salt for 6 to 8 hours

1 tablespoon minced fresh flat-leaf parsley (optional)

1 tablespoon freshly squeezed lemon juice

1 tablespoon garlic-infused olive oil

1 tablespoon reduced-sodium tamari

1 teaspoon dried thyme, well crushed between your fingers

¼ teaspoon freshly ground black pepper

2 tablespoons water, as needed

Drain the walnuts and rinse well. Put the walnuts, optional parsley, lemon juice, oil, tamari, thyme, and pepper in a food processor and process for several minutes to form a fairly smooth paste (the pâté should have some texture), stopping as needed to scrape down the container. If necessary to facilitate processing, add the water, 1 teaspoon at a time, until the desired consistency is achieved. Store in a sealed container in the refrigerator.

Curried Walnut Pâté Add ¼ teaspoon of curry powder.

Green Bean and Walnut Pâté Add 1 cup of frozen cut green beans, cooked until tender and well drained, along with ¼ teaspoon of sea salt, ¼ teaspoon of additional freshly ground black pepper, and a pinch of ground nutmeg before processing. Makes 1¼ cups.

Lentil and Walnut Pâté Add 1 cup of canned lentils, rinsed well and drained, along with ¼ teaspoon of sea salt and ¼ teaspoon of additional freshly ground black pepper before processing. Makes 1¼ cups.

Pecan Pâté Replace the walnuts with 1 cup of pecans.

TIP The walnuts can be soaked overnight or up to 72 hours in advance. Just put them in a glass container, cover with water, add a pinch of salt, cover, and let soak in the refrigerator.

Breakfast Bowls, Beverages, and Light Bites

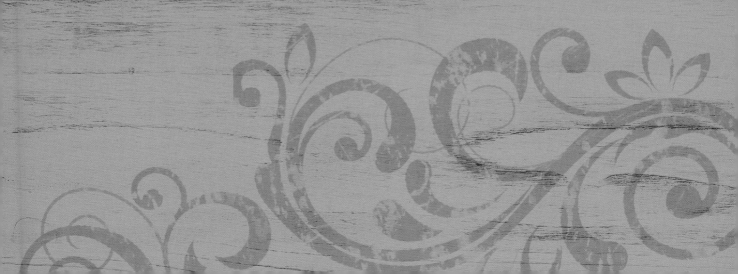

Breakfast Quinoa

MAKES 2 SERVINGS

Per serving:
143 calories
4 g protein
2 g fat (0.2 g sat)
28 g carbs
33 mg sodium
22 mg calcium
3 g fiber

If you have leftover quinoa in the fridge, you can whip up this tasty, high-protein break-fast lickety-split. It will fill you up and sustain you for hours without weighing down your tummy, and it's easy to customize with your favorite flavor combinations.

1 cup cooked quinoa (see tip, below, or table 13, page 44)

¾ cup Vanilla Almond Milk (page 47) **or low-FODMAP vanilla nondairy milk**

1 tablespoon pure maple syrup, plus more as needed

¼ heaping teaspoon ground cinnamon

Pinch sea salt

3 tablespoons chopped toasted pumpkin seeds, pecans, or walnuts (see page 53), **2 tablespoons sweetened dried cranberries, or both** (optional)

Put the quinoa, milk, maple syrup, cinnamon, and salt in a small saucepan (prefer-ably nonstick) and whisk to combine and break up any clumps of cinnamon. Bring to a boil over medium-high heat. Decrease the heat to medium and simmer, stirring frequently, until the quinoa has absorbed most of the liquid, 10 to 15 minutes. Adjust the heat as necessary to maintain a simmer, and stir more frequently toward the end when the mixture has begun to thicken. Taste and add up to 2 teaspoons of additional maple syrup if more sweetness is desired. Sprinkle with the optional seeds just before serving.

Chocolate Breakfast Quinoa Omit the cinnamon and seeds. Stir in 2 table-spoons of dark chocolate chips just before serving or sprinkle the chips over each serving.

TIP If you want to make quinoa specifically for this recipe, cook ¼ cup of quinoa in ½ cup of water per the instructions in table 13, page 44.

Creamy Oatmeal Bowls

Dessert for breakfast? Why not! Especially if it contains nuts or chocolate (yes, please!) or other sweet surprises. This creamy hot cereal is made with quick-cooking rolled oats, so it can be on the table in mere minutes. With so many options to choose from, you could serve a different version every morning of the week.

OATMEAL

1 cup Almond Milk (page 46), **Rich Almond Milk** (page 47), **Vanilla Almond Milk** (page 47), **or low-FODMAP plain or vanilla nondairy milk**

½ cup quick-cooking rolled oats

¼ cup water

Pinch sea salt

FRUIT (choose one)

1 small banana, sliced

½ cup blueberries

1 kiwifruit, peeled and diced

½ cup pineapple tidbits, fresh or packed in juice and drained

½ cup raspberries

½ cup sliced strawberries

ENRICHMENTS (choose one)

2 tablespoons dark chocolate chips

2 tablespoons chopped toasted walnuts, pecans, or peanuts

2 teaspoons no-salt-added creamy peanut butter

2 teaspoons low-FODMAP vegan butter

SWEETENER (choose one)

4 teaspoons light brown sugar

4 teaspoons pure maple syrup

4 teaspoons unbleached cane sugar

Put the milk, oats, water, and salt in a medium saucepan (preferably nonstick) and bring to a boil over medium-high heat. Decrease the heat to medium-low and simmer, stirring frequently, until thickened and the oats are cooked, 2 minutes. Serve immediately or remove from the heat, cover, and let rest for 2 to 3 minutes. Stir well. Spoon into bowls and top each serving with the fruit, enrichments, and sweetener of your choice.

MAKES 2 SERVINGS

Per serving:

218 calories

5 g protein

6 g fat (1 g sat)

36 g carbs

224 mg sodium

32 mg calcium

4 g fiber

Note: Analysis includes banana, walnuts, vegan butter, and maple syrup.

Millet Porridge

MAKES 2 SERVINGS

Per serving:

226 calories

5 g protein

9 g fat (1 g sat)

32 g carbs

51 mg sodium

0 mg calcium

6 g fiber

Despite being light and easy to digest, millet is a powerhouse of nutrition. Naturally gluten-free, it's high in protein, fiber, B-complex vitamins, and important minerals and amino acids. This porridge takes a bit of time to cook, so make it on leisurely mornings. It's best served fresh and hot, as cooked millet tends to dry out and harden when refrigerated.

⅓ **cup hulled millet**

¾ **cup water**

½ **cup Almond Milk** (page 46), **Rich Almond Milk** (page 47), **Vanilla Almond Milk** (page 47), **or low-FODMAP plain or vanilla nondairy milk**

2 **teaspoons low-FODMAP vegan butter or coconut oil**

½ **teaspoon vanilla extract**

¼ **teaspoon ground cinnamon**

Pinch sea salt

2 **tablespoons sweetened dried cranberries, whole or chopped**

2 **tablespoons chopped toasted pecans** (see page 53)

Pure maple syrup, brown sugar, or unbleached cane sugar, as needed

Put the millet in a small saucepan (preferably nonstick). Add the water, milk, butter, vanilla extract, cinnamon, and salt and bring to a boil over medium-high heat. Decrease the heat to low, cover, and cook, stirring occasionally, until the liquid is absorbed and the millet is soft and tender, about 35 minutes. Add the cranberries and beat vigorously until they are evenly incorporated and the millet is creamy. Spoon into bowls. Sprinkle each serving with half the pecans and drizzle with maple syrup to taste. Serve immediately.

Maple–Peanut Butter Oatmeal

MAKES 1 SERVING

Per serving:

145 calories

5 g protein

2 g fat (0.3 g sat)

29 g carbs

48 mg sodium

18 mg calcium

5 g fiber

Powdered peanut butter infuses this oatmeal with extra flavor and protein but with almost no additional calories or fat compared to regular peanut butter. In mere minutes, you can have a power-packed, low-FODMAP breakfast that will keep you satisfied for hours.

¼ **cup quick-cooking rolled oats**

¾ **cup water**

2 **heaping teaspoons powdered peanut butter or peanut flour** (see box and tip, page 67)

1 **tablespoon pure maple syrup**

Pinch sea salt

½ **teaspoon low-FODMAP vegan butter** (optional)

Put the oats in a small saucepan (preferably nonstick). Add the water, powdered peanut butter, maple syrup, and salt. Bring to a boil over medium-high heat. Decrease the heat to medium-low and simmer, stirring frequently, until thickened and the oats are cooked, 2 minutes. Serve immediately or remove from the heat, cover, and let rest for 2 to 3 minutes. Stir well. Spoon into a bowl and swirl in the optional vegan butter.

Chocolate–Peanut Butter Oatmeal Replace the powdered peanut butter with 2 heaping teaspoons of chocolate powdered peanut butter and replace the maple syrup with 2 heaping teaspoons of unbleached cane sugar. If you use plain powdered peanut butter or peanut flour, whisk in 2 teaspoons of unsweetened cocoa powder and replace the maple syrup with 1 tablespoon of unbleached cane sugar. Add more water or sugar as needed.

Strawberry-Coconut Oatmeal Add 2 to 3 tablespoons of chopped fresh or freeze-dried strawberries and 1 teaspoon of unsweetened shredded dried coconut before or after cooking.

TIP If you're using unsweetened peanut flour, add more maple syrup or unbleached cane sugar to taste (see box, below).

FAT-REDUCED POWDERED PEANUT BUTTER AND PEANUT FLOUR

Powdered peanut butter and peanut flour are made from real roasted peanuts with the fat removed, resulting in a product that's much lower in fat (around 1.5 grams rather than 16 grams per 2 tablespoons) and calories (around 45 calories versus 200 calories per 2 tablespoons) than regular peanut butter. Although powdered peanut butter and peanut flour can be reconstituted with water to make a spread, the texture and flavor really shine when the powder or flour is used in recipes. Look for organic powdered peanut butter and flour (see Resources, page 133). Be sure to purchase fat-reduced peanut flour, as some brands contain the full amount of fat.

Be aware that most brands of powdered peanut butter contain cane sugar or another sweetener, such as coconut sugar (which hasn't been tested yet for FODMAPs) or stevia, which is FODMAP-free, so additional sweetener often isn't needed. If you use powdered peanut butter that contains coconut sugar, try it in small quantities over two to three days and monitor your symptoms. If it's well tolerated, you can use it safely. Note that peanut flour isn't sweetened, so if you use it instead of sweetened powdered peanut butter in oatmeal, smoothies, or other sweet recipes, add 1 heaping teaspoon of pure maple syrup or unbleached cane sugar for every tablespoon of peanut flour used.

Vanilla Tapioca Pudding

MAKES 4 SERVINGS

Per serving:

161 calories

0 g protein

8 g fat (8 g sat)

22 g carbs

146 mg sodium

0 mg calcium

0 g fiber

Chewy, round tapioca pearls are made from low-FODMAP tapioca starch. The fun-to-eat pearls, which come in assorted sizes and colors, including white, brown, and even pastels, are commonly used in beverages, bubble teas, puddings, and other desserts. This ultra-creamy tapioca pudding makes a delicious breakfast or after-dinner dessert, served plain or topped with low-FODMAP fresh fruit or berries.

⅓ cup small tapioca pearls

1½ cups Vanilla Almond Milk (page 47) or low-FODMAP vanilla nondairy milk

1 can (13.5 ounces; 1⅔ cups) light coconut milk

⅓ cup unbleached cane sugar or pure maple syrup

1 teaspoon vanilla extract

¼ teaspoon sea salt

Ground cinnamon, or 4 teaspoons unsweetened shredded dried coconut

Put the tapioca pearls in a deep, large saucepan (preferably nonstick). Add the almond milk and set aside for 1 to 2 hours to let the tapioca pearls rehydrate and soften.

Add the coconut milk, sugar, vanilla extract, and salt and bring to a boil over medium-high heat. Decrease the heat to medium and cook, stirring occasionally, until the tapioca pearls are tender and transparent and the pudding has thickened, 15 to 20 minutes (it will thicken further as it cools). Adjust the heat as necessary to maintain a gentle simmer, and stir more frequently toward the end when the pudding has begun to thicken.

Spoon evenly into four small custard cups. Serve at room temperature or cover tightly and chill thoroughly before serving. Sprinkle with cinnamon before serving.

Dark Chocolate Tapioca Pudding Replace the Vanilla Almond Milk with Chocolate Almond Milk (page 47) or other low-FODMAP chocolate nondairy milk. Increase the sugar to 6 tablespoons. Whisk in 4 tablespoons of unsweetened cocoa powder and cook the pudding as directed. Omit the cinnamon. If desired, garnish each serving with 1 teaspoon of unsweetened shredded dried coconut or mini chocolate chips.

Milk Chocolate Tapioca Pudding Cook the pudding as directed. Remove from the heat and stir in ¼ cup of dark chocolate chips until melted and evenly combined. Omit the cinnamon. If desired, garnish each serving with 1 teaspoon of unsweetened shredded dried coconut.

Strawberry Tapioca Pudding Increase the sugar to 6 tablespoons. Cook the pudding as directed. Remove from the heat and stir in ½ cup of coarsely chopped fresh strawberries until evenly combined.

Basmati Rice Pudding

Cardamom adds a hint of the exotic and coconut milk and almond milk impart creamy richness to this traditional, go-to comfort food.

⅓ cup white basmati rice

⅔ cup water

1 can (13.5 ounces; 1⅔ cups) light coconut milk

¾ cup Vanilla Almond Milk (page 47) or low-FODMAP vanilla nondairy milk

⅓ cup unbleached cane sugar

¼ teaspoon ground cardamom

¼ teaspoon sea salt

¼ cup sweetened dried cranberries, chopped

8 teaspoons chopped toasted pecans (see page 53; optional)

MAKES 4 SERVINGS

Per serving:

153 calories

1 g protein

5 g fat (4 g sat)

26 g carbs

156 mg sodium

0 mg calcium

1 g fiber

Put the rice in a deep, large saucepan (preferably nonstick). Add the water and bring to a boil over medium-high heat. Decrease the heat to low, cover, and cook until the rice is tender and the water is absorbed, 15 to 18 minutes. Remove from the heat and let rest, covered, for 5 to 10 minutes. Add the coconut milk, almond milk, sugar, cardamom, and salt and whisk to combine and break up any clumps of cardamom. Bring to a boil over medium-high heat. Decrease the heat to medium and cook, stirring frequently, until the mixture is thick, 25 to 30 minutes. Adjust the heat as necessary to maintain a gentle simmer, and stir more frequently toward the end when the pudding has begun to thicken.

Remove from the heat and stir in the cranberries. Spoon evenly into four small custard cups. Let cool slightly. Serve warm or cover tightly and chill thoroughly before serving. Sprinkle each serving with 2 teaspoons of the optional pecans before serving.

Dark Chocolate Rice Pudding Omit the cardamom, cranberries, and pecans. Replace the Vanilla Almond Milk with 1 cup of Chocolate Almond Milk (page 47) or other low-FODMAP chocolate nondairy milk. Increase the sugar to 6 tablespoons. Whisk in 4 tablespoons of unsweetened cocoa powder and cook the pudding as directed. If desired, garnish each serving with 1 teaspoon of unsweetened shredded dried coconut or mini chocolate chips.

Milk Chocolate Rice Pudding Omit the cardamom, cranberries, and pecans. Cook the pudding as directed. Remove from the heat and stir in ¼ cup of dark chocolate chips until melted and evenly combined. If desired, garnish each serving with 1 teaspoon of unsweetened shredded dried coconut.

Strawberry Rice Pudding Omit the cranberries. Increase the sugar to 6 tablespoons. Cook the pudding as directed. Remove from the heat and stir in ½ cup of coarsely chopped fresh strawberries until evenly combined.

Pumpkin Pie Mousse

MAKES 2 SERVINGS

Per serving:

224 calories

6 g protein

8 g fat (1 g sat)

33 g carbs

7 mg sodium

43 mg calcium

4 g fiber

I'm a firm believer in dessert for breakfast, especially if it's wholesome but tastes decadent. Of course, this light, silky mousse also makes a delicious snack or after-dinner dessert.

1 firm banana, broken into pieces

½ cup canned pumpkin purée or sweet potato purée

¼ cup Almond Milk (page 46), **Rich Almond Milk** (page 47), **low-FODMAP plain nondairy milk, or light coconut milk**

2 tablespoons no-salt-added creamy peanut butter

2 tablespoons pure maple syrup

½ teaspoon ground cinnamon

¼ teaspoon ground ginger

⅛ teaspoon ground nutmeg

Pinch ground cloves or allspice

Put all the ingredients in a blender or food processor and process until smooth. Spoon evenly into two small custard cups. Serve immediately or cover tightly and chill for up to 3 hours.

Pecan Pie Mousse Sprinkle 1 heaping tablespoon of chopped toasted pecans (see page 53) over each serving.

> **TIP** Don't know what to do with the remaining pumpkin purée? Just freeze it in half-cup portions. That way, you can defrost it overnight in the fridge and be ready to make this scrumptious mousse first thing in the morning. Alternatively, use leftover pumpkin purée in a Pumpkin Pie Smoothie (page 73).

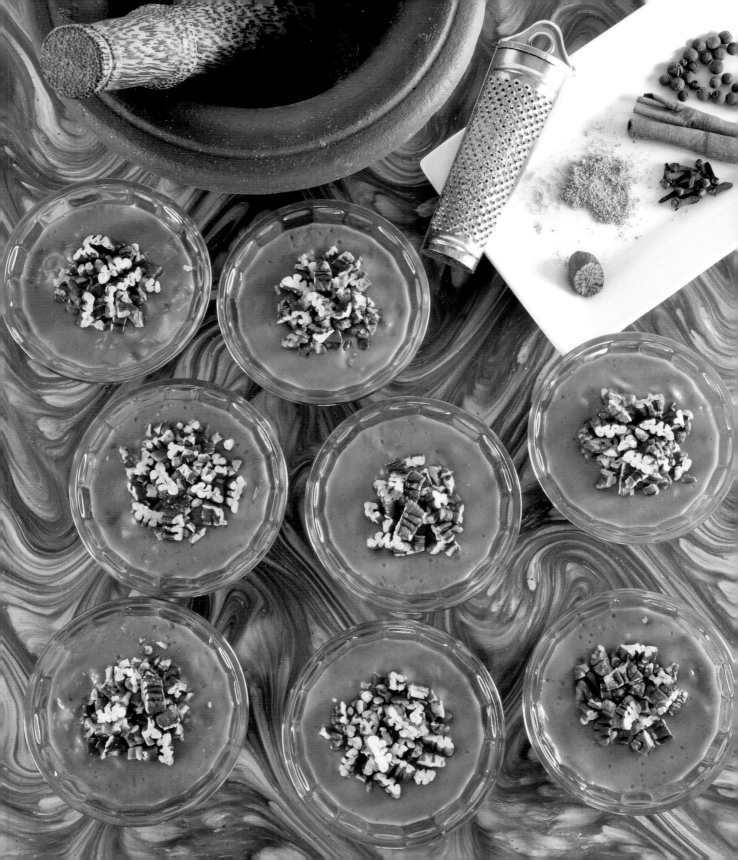

Maple-Vanilla Soft Serve

MAKES 1 SERVING

Per serving:

121 calories

1 g protein

0 g fat (0 g sat)

30 g carbs

2 mg sodium

10 mg calcium

3 g fiber

By blending a frozen banana with a little maple syrup and vanilla extract, you can instantly create a low-FODMAP, dairy-free, soft-serve ice cream for a fun, light breakfast or sweet snack or dessert. It's a nutritious, creamy, guilt-free treat that's ideal whenever you're craving something comforting. If you keep a few ripe bananas in the freezer, you can make this soft serve at the spur of the moment.

1 frozen small banana, broken into pieces
1½ teaspoons pure maple syrup
½ teaspoon vanilla extract

Put all the ingredients in a food processor and process for 30 seconds. Scrape down the container and process until smooth, 30 to 60 seconds longer. Serve immediately.

Maple-Vanilla Banana Pudding Replace the frozen banana with 1 firm fresh banana and proceed with the recipe as directed.

Peanut Butter–Fudge Soft Serve Replace the maple syrup with 2 teaspoons of unbleached cane sugar. Add 2 teaspoons of creamy peanut butter and 1½ teaspoons of unsweetened cocoa powder and proceed with the recipe as directed.

Strawberry–Poppy Seed Soft Serve Replace the maple syrup with an equal amount of unbleached cane sugar. Add 2 hulled fresh strawberries and ½ teaspoon of black poppy seeds and proceed with the recipe as directed.

Peanut Butter–Banana Instant Breakfast Drink

On days when nothing sounds appealing except liquids, this go-to light beverage will hit the spot and lift your spirits. Use chocolate powdered peanut butter for an extra-special treat.

1 cup Vanilla Almond Milk (page 47) **or low-FODMAP vanilla nondairy milk, or 1 cup cold water plus 1 tablespoon almond butter or tahini and ½ teaspoon vanilla extract**

1 frozen small banana, broken into pieces

2 heaping tablespoons chocolate or plain powdered peanut butter or peanut flour (see box, page 67, and tip, below)

MAKES 1 SERVING

Per serving:

149 calories

6 g protein

5 g fat (0.1 g sat)

102 g carbs

97 mg sodium

10 mg calcium

5 g fiber

Put all the ingredients in a high-powered blender and process until smooth.

Pumpkin Pie Smoothie Use plain powdered peanut butter. Add 2 tablespoons of canned pumpkin purée, 1 tablespoon of pure maple syrup, ½ teaspoon of ground cinnamon, ¼ teaspoon of ground ginger, ⅛ teaspoon of ground nutmeg, and a pinch of ground allspice.

Snickerdoodle Smoothie Use plain powdered peanut butter and add ¼ teaspoon of ground cinnamon and a pinch of ground nutmeg. Sprinkle with additional cinnamon before serving.

TIP If you use unsweetened peanut flour, add unbleached cane sugar or pure maple syrup to taste (see box, page 67). If you use plain powdered peanut butter or peanut flour and want a chocolate-flavored drink, add 2 teaspoons of unsweetened cocoa powder and additional sugar to taste.

No-Bake Peanut Butter Granola Bars

MAKES 8 BARS

Per bar:

290 calories

8 g protein

18 g fat (5 g sat)

27 g carbs

3 mg sodium

32 mg calcium

5 g fiber

These gently sweetened, high-protein granola bars are soft and delicate, unlike the often dry, cardboard-like, commercial granola bars or fruit-and-nut bars. These tender treats are filling and perfect for breakfast or a snack on the run. Plus, they're loaded with chocolate chips and don't require any baking. What could be better?

¾ cup no-salt-added creamy peanut butter (see tip)

3 tablespoons pure maple syrup

2 tablespoons rice syrup (see tip)

1 teaspoon vanilla extract

Pinch sea salt (optional)

1 cup quick-cooking rolled oats

¼ cup mini chocolate chips

¼ cup sweetened dried cranberries, chopped (optional)

¼ cup walnuts, finely chopped (optional)

3 tablespoons unsweetened finely shredded dried coconut

Lightly oil an 8-inch square baking pan.

Put the peanut butter, maple syrup, rice syrup, vanilla extract, and optional salt in a medium bowl. Stir until smooth and well combined. Add the rolled oats, chocolate chips, optional cranberries, optional walnuts, and coconut. Stir to combine, then use your hands to knead the mixture well until all the ingredients are evenly distributed. The mixture will be very stiff, but the more you knead it, the better it will hold together.

Press the mixture very firmly and evenly into the oiled baking pan using your hands. Cover with plastic wrap, pressing it directly on the mixture. Cover the pan with foil or a lid. Refrigerate for at least 4 hours before slicing and serving. Tightly wrap leftovers and store in the refrigerator or freezer.

TIP Rice syrup is a light, mild, very sticky sweetener. For the best results, don't substitute any other sweetener for it in this recipe. To make the syrup easier to remove, oil the measuring cup or spoon before measuring the syrup. Be sure to use very smooth, very creamy peanut butter, preferably from a jar rather than the self-grinding machine at the store, which will produce a thicker, coarser grind. The drier, thicker, and coarser the peanut butter, the drier and more crumbly the granola bars will be.

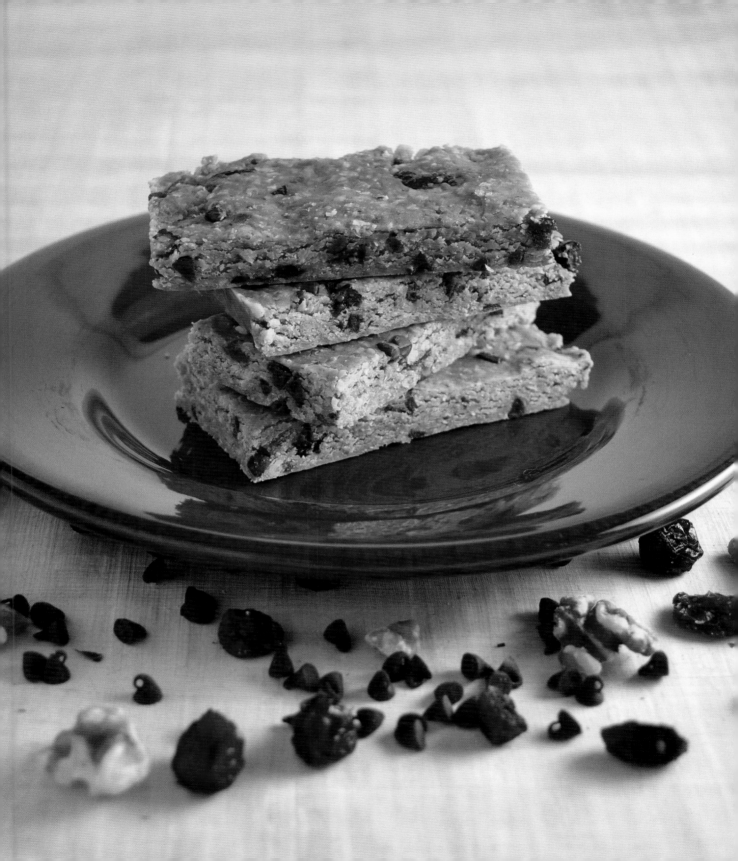

Berry Good Smoothie

MAKES 1 SERVING

Per serving:

196 calories

6 g protein

2 g fat (0.1 g sat)

42 g carbs

171 mg sodium

12 mg calcium

5 g fiber

This smoothie is lusciously thick and satisfying. With the smaller portions of fruit, it handily stays within the low-FODMAP guidelines for one serving. The powdered peanut butter adds a welcome boost of protein and creaminess while keeping the smoothie low in fat.

1 cup Vanilla Almond Milk (page 47), **low-FODMAP vanilla nondairy milk, or 1 cup cold water plus 1 tablespoon almond butter or peanut butter**

½ frozen banana, broken into pieces

½ cup frozen blueberries or raspberries, or 6 frozen strawberries

1 tablespoon pure maple syrup

2 heaping tablespoons chocolate or plain powdered peanut butter or peanut flour (see box, page 67, and tip, below)

Put all the ingredients in a high-powered blender and process until smooth.

Berry Good Green Smoothie Add ¼ to ½ cup of baby spinach, lightly packed, before processing.

Chocolate-Covered Strawberry Smoothie Replace the milk with 1 cup of Chocolate Almond Milk (page 47) or low-FODMAP chocolate nondairy milk and use frozen strawberries for the berries.

Pineapple Smoothie Replace the berries with ½ cup of frozen pineapple chunks.

Pineapple-Berry Smoothie Decrease the berries to ¼ cup or 3 frozen strawberries and add ¼ cup of frozen pineapple chunks.

TIP If you use unsweetened peanut flour, add more maple syrup or unbleached cane sugar to taste (see box, page 67). If you use plain powdered peanut butter or peanut flour and want a chocolate-flavored smoothie, add 2 teaspoons of unsweetened cocoa powder and additional maple syrup or sugar to taste.

Crispy Rice Treats with Chocolate Drizzle

These eye-catching squares are surprisingly low in fat yet are decadently delicious. They make a pleasing snack, quick breakfast (alongside a serving of suitable fruit), fun dessert, or a sensational party or potluck contribution. To keep the FODMAPs low, have just one square at a sitting.

½ **cup rice syrup** (see tip, page 74)

4 tablespoons no-salt-added creamy peanut butter or almond butter

1 tablespoon coconut oil

1 teaspoon vanilla extract

Pinch sea salt (optional)

4 cups crispy rice cereal

⅓ **cup dark chocolate chips**

MAKES 16 SQUARES

Per square:

116 calories

2 g protein

4 g fat (2 g sat)

17 g carbs

63 mg sodium

2 mg calcium

1 g fiber

Oil an 8-inch square baking pan.

Put the rice syrup, peanut butter, oil, vanilla extract, and optional salt in a large saucepan (preferably nonstick). Heat over medium heat, stirring frequently, until the peanut butter and syrup are soft and warm and the ingredients are well combined, about 3 minutes. Remove from the heat and stir in the cereal until evenly combined. Transfer to the oiled baking pan and use a silicone spatula or your hands to distribute the mixture evenly (it will be sticky). Lightly oil the back of a metal spatula and press down on the flat blade with your hands to firmly and evenly pack the mixture into the pan.

Melt the chocolate chips in a microwave, double boiler, or small saucepan (preferably nonstick) over very low heat. Drizzle the melted chocolate in a random pattern over the cereal mixture using a spoon. Refrigerate for 30 minutes before cutting into squares. Store in a tightly sealed container in the refrigerator or at room temperature.

Breakfast Scramble

MAKES 2 SERVINGS

Per serving:

129 calories

10 g protein

9 g fat (2 g sat)

4 g carbs

18 mg sodium

237 mg calcium

2 g fiber

This union of tofu and vegetables makes a tasty savory morning meal or light supper. For a special brunch, serve the scramble with sliced tomatoes, Tempeh Bacon (page 49), and gluten-free crackers or toasted 100% sourdough spelt bread, millet bread, or gluten-free vegan bread.

TIP Scrambles will turn out more tender and moist if the tofu used is on the softer side. For that reason, use firm or extra-firm (rather than super-firm) tofu in this recipe and don't press it.

2 teaspoons garlic-infused olive oil

¼ teaspoon asafetida (see page 29; optional)

¼ cup diced red or green bell pepper

¼ cup shredded carrot

¼ cup thinly sliced chives or scallion greens, or 4 teaspoons dried chives

¼ teaspoon ground turmeric

8 ounces firm or extra-firm tofu, rinsed, patted dry, and crumbled (see tip)

2 teaspoons nutritional yeast flakes (optional but highly recommended)

2 tablespoons minced fresh flat-leaf parsley or cilantro, or 2 teaspoons dried parsley

10 pitted kalamata, oil-cured, or black olives, sliced or chopped (optional)

¼ teaspoon black salt (see box, below; optional)

Sea salt

Freshly ground black pepper

Put the oil in a medium skillet (preferably nonstick) and heat over medium-high heat. When hot, add the optional asafetida and let it sizzle for about 30 seconds. Add bell pepper, carrot, chives, and turmeric and cook, stirring occasionally, for 4 minutes. Add the tofu and optional nutritional yeast and stir until well combined. Decrease the heat to medium and cook, stirring occasionally, until the tofu is hot and lightly browned, 8 to 10 minutes. Add the parsley, optional olives, and optional black salt and stir until evenly distributed. Season with sea salt and pepper to taste.

Note: Analysis doesn't include sea salt or freshly ground black pepper to taste.

A VEGAN TASTE OF EGGS

Black salt, also known as *kala namak* or *sanchal,* is a type of Indian volcanic rock salt commonly used in the cuisines of India, Pakistan, and other Asian countries. Because it contains iron and other minerals, it's actually pinkish-gray rather than black and has a very distinctive sulfurous taste and aroma that has been compared to hard-boiled egg yolks. Including black salt in scrambled tofu and similar dishes will impart an authentic egg-like taste. Look for black salt in Indian markets and online.

8

Dinner Buffet

Indian-Style Chard, Potatoes, and Carrots

MAKES 4 SERVINGS

Per serving:

234 calories

7 g protein

9 g fat (6 g sat)

34 g carbs

276 mg sodium

115 mg calcium

7 g fiber

This mildly spiced dish features three common low-FODMAP vegetables that are available year-round. If you want to kick the heat up a notch, add a pinch of cayenne or crushed red pepper flakes along with the other spices, or stir in a little Mild Hot Chile Paste (page 54) with the lemon juice in the last step.

2 tablespoons coconut oil

2 teaspoons garlic-infused olive oil

1 tablespoon peeled and grated fresh ginger

2 teaspoons ground cumin, or 1 teaspoon whole cumin seeds

1 teaspoon ground fenugreek

1 teaspoon ground turmeric

3 large carrots, peeled and thinly sliced

2 large potatoes, peeled and diced

1 pound rainbow Swiss chard, stems trimmed, leaves and ribs coarsely chopped

½ cup water

½ teaspoon sea salt, plus more as needed

¾ cup no-salt-added chickpeas, rinsed well and drained (optional)

1 tablespoon freshly squeezed lemon juice

Put the coconut oil and garlic-infused oil in a large saucepan (preferably nonstick) over medium heat. When hot, add the ginger, cumin, fenugreek, and turmeric and cook, stirring constantly, for 1 minute. Add the carrots and potatoes and stir to coat with the oil and spices. Cook, stirring frequently, for 5 minutes. Add the chard and cook, stirring constantly, until the leaves are wilted, about 5 minutes. Add the water and salt and stir to combine. Cover and cook, stirring occasionally, for 10 minutes. Add the optional chickpeas and stir to combine. Cover and cook, stirring occasionally, until the potatoes and carrots are very tender, 5 to 10 minutes longer. Season with the lemon juice and additional salt to taste.

Coconut-Curry Tofu and Veggie Stir-Fry

This gently seasoned stir-fry is an excellent dinner staple, and leftovers make a welcome lunch. For an even more filling dish, serve the stir-fry over cooked quinoa, rice, or gluten-free pasta. Feel free to swap out the vegetables with your low-FODMAP favorites.

MAKES 4 SERVINGS

Per serving:

330 calories

23 g protein

22 g fat (10 g sat)

11 g carbs

489 mg sodium

138 mg calcium

4 g fiber

1 pound superfirm or extra-firm tofu, pressed (see page 28) **and cut into strips about 2 inches long, ½ inch wide, and ¼ inch thick**

2 tablespoons reduced-sodium tamari

1 tablespoon coconut oil

¼ teaspoon asafetida (see page 29; optional)

¼ cup raw or toasted pumpkin seeds (see page 53)

2 tablespoons peeled and grated fresh ginger

2 carrots, peeled and thinly sliced on the diagonal

2 small zucchini, halved lengthwise and thinly sliced on the diagonal

1 head baby bok choy, sliced crosswise on the diagonal

1 tablespoon curry powder

¼ teaspoon freshly ground black pepper

1 cup light coconut milk

¼ cup chopped fresh cilantro or flat-leaf parsley, packed

Sea salt

Mild Hot Chile Paste (page 54)**, Mild Hot Sauce** (page 54)**, Tabasco, or cayenne** (optional)

Put the tofu in a medium bowl, sprinkle with the tamari, and toss gently to coat each piece evenly. Set aside to marinate while you prepare the vegetables.

Put the oil in a large skillet or wide saucepan (preferably nonstick) over medium-high heat. When hot, add the optional asafetida and let it sizzle for about 30 seconds. Add the pumpkin seeds and ginger and stir to combine. Add the carrots and cook, stirring frequently, until slightly softened, 5 to 10 minutes. Add the zucchini and bok choy and cook, stirring almost constantly, until all the vegetables are tender, about 8 minutes. Add the curry powder and pepper and stir until evenly distributed. Add the tofu, coconut milk, and cilantro and gently stir to combine. Season with salt and optional chile paste to taste. Decrease the heat to low, cover, and cook, stirring occasionally, until heated through and the flavors have blended, about 5 minutes.

Roasted Veggies with Dilled Lemon-Caper Sauce

MAKES 4 SERVINGS

Per serving:

290 calories

6 g protein

14 g fat (2 g sat)

35 g carbs

192 mg sodium

74 mg calcium

7 g fiber

This recipe is a turn-to staple not only because it's irresistibly delicious and wholesome, but also because it practically makes itself. Once the veggies are prepped and in the oven, set a timer and go read a book for a while. The sauce takes just a minute to put together, and the whole dish is so spectacularly impressive, no one would guess how easy it is.

VEGETABLES

1 pound baby potatoes (a mix of red, gold, and purple or a single color), **scrubbed**

1 bag (1 pound) **baby carrots, or 1 pound parsnips, peeled and cut into 2-inch pieces, or 1 pound mixed baby carrots and parsnips**

1 tablespoon basil-infused, herb-infused, or plain extra-virgin olive oil

1 tablespoon garlic-infused olive oil

Sea salt

Freshly ground black pepper

2 zucchini, sliced into 1-inch-thick pieces, 1 eggplant cut into 1-inch cubes, 8 ounces green beans or haricot verts, trimmed (1½ to 2 cups), or 3 heads baby bok choy, trimmed and sliced in half crosswise

1 red bell pepper, cut into large squares

DILLED LEMON-CAPER SAUCE

3 tablespoons vegan mayonnaise

1 tablespoon freshly squeezed lemon juice

1 tablespoon dried dill weed

1½ teaspoons dried tarragon, crushed between your fingers

1 teaspoon small capers, well drained

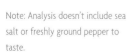 **TIP** If you're fortunate to have fresh dill on hand, use 3 tablespoons of fresh dill in the sauce instead of the dried dill weed, and sprinkle a little extra fresh dill over each serving for an even more beautiful presentation.

Preheat the oven to 425 degrees F.

If the potatoes are large, cut them in half. Put the potatoes and carrots in a large roasting pan. Add the basil-infused oil and garlic-infused oil. Sprinkle generously with salt and pepper as desired. Stir until the vegetables are evenly coated with the oil and seasonings and spread into a single layer. Bake for 20 minutes. Remove from the oven and stir. Add the zucchini and bell pepper, stir well to coat with the oil, and spread into a single layer. Bake for 15 minutes. Remove from the oven, stir, spread into a single layer, and bake for 10 minutes longer, or until the vegetables are dark brown in spots and the potatoes are fork-tender.

When the vegetables are almost done roasting, prepare the sauce. Put all the sauce ingredients in a small bowl and stir until evenly combined. Top each serving of the roasted vegetables with a dollop of the sauce or pass the sauce at the table.

Roasted Veggie and Legume Salad Prepare the roasted vegetables as directed. Transfer to a large bowl. Add 1 can (15 ounces) of lentils or 1 cup of

Note: Analysis doesn't include sea salt or freshly ground pepper to taste.

canned chickpeas, rinsed well and drained, and toss gently to combine. Top each serving with a dollop of the Dilled Lemon-Caper Sauce or stir the sauce into the salad until evenly distributed. Alternatively, replace the sauce with ⅓ cup of Classic Vinaigrette and Marinade or one of the variations (page 116).

Variation   Replace the Dilled Lemon-Caper Sauce with ¼ cup of Remoulade Sauce (page 84), Sriracha Mayo (page 56), Sriracha-Mustard Mayo (page 56), or Yum-Yum Sauce (page 108).

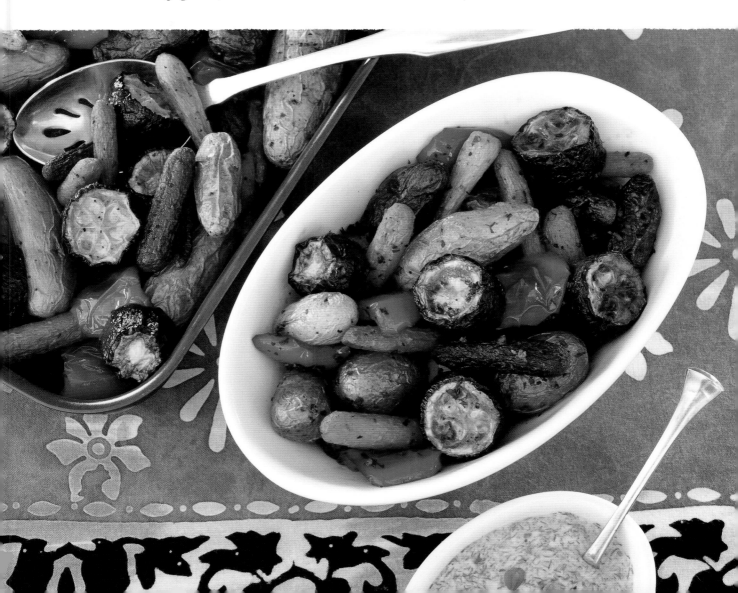

Tortilla Pull-Aparts

MAKES 2 SERVINGS

Per serving:

575 calories

11 g protein

39 g fat (4 g sat)

48 g carbs

689 mg sodium

156 mg calcium

9 g fiber

See photo, page 86

Tortilla pull-aparts are a fun-to-eat cross between burrito bowls, nachos, and an overloaded pizza, but they're also quick and healthy one-plate meals. If you have leftovers of any of the bases sitting in the fridge, this is a great way to use them up. Of course, in the event this dish becomes a staple in your house (as it has in mine), you might want to prepare a base or two specifically to use in this recipe. Neat-and-tidy types can eat the pull-aparts with a knife and fork, but if you don't mind making a mess, just dig in with your hands and pull them apart.

REMOULADE SAUCE

3 tablespoons vegan mayo

1 tablespoon Good-to-Your-Gut Sriracha Sauce (page 56) **or tomato purée, plus more as needed, or 1 teaspoon Mild Hot Chile Paste** (page 54)

2 teaspoons yellow mustard

Pinch smoked paprika (optional)

Tabasco or Mild Hot Sauce (page 54)

TORTILLAS

2 large brown rice tortillas

BASE (choose one)

4 ounces Barbecued Tempeh Short Ribs (page 88)

6 ounces Barbecued Tofu Short Ribs (page 88)

6 ounces Chickenless Chicken (page 52)

6 tablespoons Chive Cheese Spread (page 60)

4 ounces Ginger-Glazed Tempeh Filets (page 87)

1 cup Greek Tofu Feta (page 48), **crumbled**

6 tablespoons Green Bean and Walnut Pâté (page 62)

4 ounces Herbed Tempeh Nuggets (page 51)

6 tablespoons I Can't Believe It's Not Cheese Spread (page 60)

6 ounces Lemon-Pepper Tofu (page 50)

6 tablespoons Lentil and Walnut Pâté (page 62)

6 tablespoons Lentil Hummus (page 61)

6 tablespoons Lentil-Chickpea Hummus (page 61)

6 ounces Maple-Miso Tofu (page 50)

1 cup seitan strips or cubes

4 ounces Tempeh Bacon (page 49)

4 ounces Teriyaki Tempeh (page 90)

6 ounces Tofu Bacon Strips or Slabs (page 49)

⅔ cup shredded vegan cheese

6 tablespoons Walnut Pâté (page 62)

VEGGIES

2 cups baby spinach, firmly packed

1 cup shredded carrots

1 small red bell pepper, diced

¼ cup thinly sliced scallion greens, or 10 pitted kalamata or oil-cured olives, chopped or sliced

2 mini cucumbers, or ½ small English cucumber, thinly sliced

2 cups baby arugula, packed

2 cups mesclun, packed

Fresh basil leaves, torn, or thinly sliced scallion greens (optional)

Note: Analysis includes Walnut Pâté (page 62).

Preheat the oven to 400 degrees F.

To make the sauce, put the mayonnaise, sriracha sauce, mustard, and optional smoked paprika in a small bowl and stir or whisk until smooth and well combined. Season with Tabasco to taste. For a thinner sauce, add more sriracha sauce, tomato purée, or water, 1 teaspoon at a time, until the desired consistency is achieved.

To make the pull-aparts, put the tortillas on a large sheet of parchment paper or on a parchment-lined baking sheet. If using a spread, pâté, or hummus, put half the mixture in the center of each tortilla and spread it out in a circle as best as possible, leaving a one- to two-inch margin. If using Chickenless Chicken, Greek Tofu Feta, Lemon-Pepper Tofu, Maple-Miso Tofu, seitan, or cheese, arrange in a single layer, leaving a one- to two-inch margin. Top with the spinach, covering the base as completely as possible and extending into the margin. Next, layer on the carrots, bell pepper, and scallion greens, in that order. Carefully transfer the tortillas along with the parchment paper directly to the oven rack or put the baking sheet on the oven rack and bake until the tortillas are dark brown and crisp around the edges and the vegetables are cooked, about 18 minutes.

Carefully transfer the tortillas to plates using a metal spatula (bring the plates to the tortillas, rather than the other way around, to avoid dropping them). Arrange the cucumber slices in a single layer in concentric circles over the vegetables. Top with the arugula and mesclun. Scatter the optional basil leaves over the mesclun. Drizzle or dollop the sauce evenly over the top. Serve immediately.

Variation Replace the Remoulade Sauce with 4 to 6 tablespoons of Dilled Lemon-Caper Sauce (page 82), I Can't Believe It's Not Cheese Sauce (page 60), Lemon-Tahini Dressing (page 115), Sriracha Dressing (page 56), Sriracha Mayo (page 56), Sriracha-Mustard Mayo (page 56), or Yum-Yum Sauce (page 108).

TIP If you have leftover cooked vegetables, use them to replace all or part of the spinach.

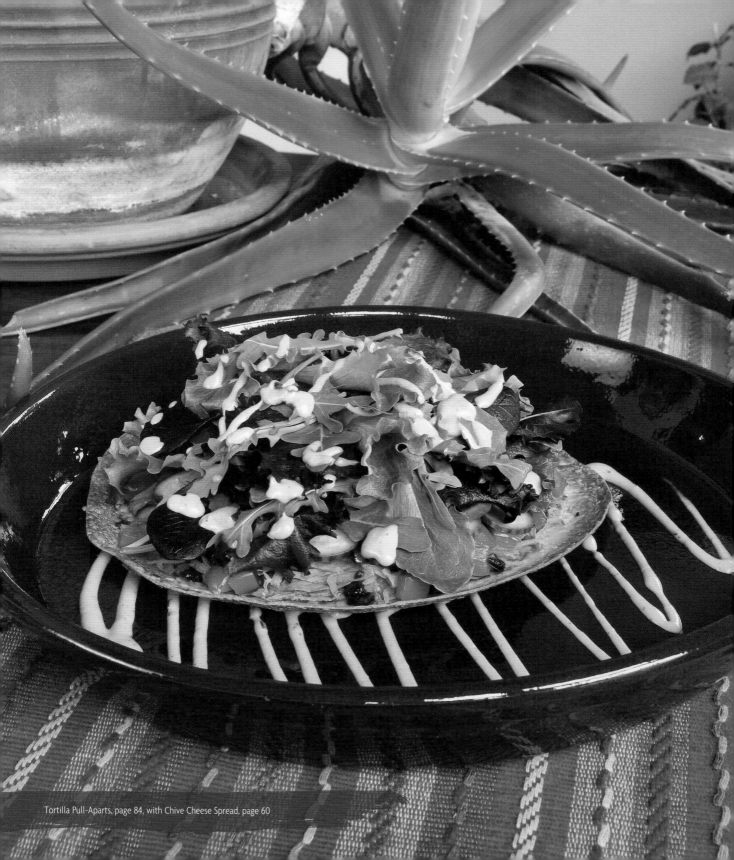

Tortilla Pull-Aparts, page 84, with Chive Cheese Spread, page 60

Ginger-Glazed Tempeh Filets

This is a very quick and easy way to infuse tempeh with deep, rich flavor. Ginger imparts a spicy kick, and maple syrup, tamari, and citrus juice balance out the bite. Serve these filets alongside rice, mashed or baked potatoes (see page 102), or polenta (see table 13, page 44). Add a steamed vegetable and/or salad and call it dinner!

½ cup water

3 tablespoons pure maple syrup

2 tablespoons reduced-sodium tamari

1½ tablespoons freshly squeezed lemon or lime juice

1 tablespoon garlic-infused olive oil

2 teaspoons peeled and grated fresh ginger, or 1 teaspoon powdered ginger

Pinch sea salt (optional)

Pinch cayenne (optional)

8 ounces tempeh, cut crosswise into ½-inch-thick filets

MAKES 14 FILETS, 4 SERVINGS

Per serving:
189 calories
12 g protein
10 g fat (2 g sat)
17 g carbs
303 mg sodium
72 mg calcium
0 g fiber

Put the water, maple syrup, tamari, lemon juice, oil, ginger, optional salt, and optional cayenne in a deep, wide saucepan or skillet (preferably nonstick) and stir to combine. Add the tempeh and gently stir to coat the pieces all over. Bring to a simmer over medium-high heat. Decrease the heat to medium and cook, gently turning the pieces over occasionally and adjusting the heat as necessary to maintain a simmer, until the liquid has cooked off or been absorbed and the tempeh is well browned on both sides, about 20 minutes.

Barbecued Tempeh Short Ribs

MAKES 4 SERVINGS

Per serving:

163 calories

13 g protein

6 g fat (1 g sat)

17 g carbs

199 mg sodium

70 mg calcium

1 g fiber

Barbecued tempeh strips make for some hearty eating. The strips are marinated in a zesty low-FODMAP sauce and then baked to create moist and tender meatless barbecued short ribs. Serve them with mashed or baked potatoes (see page 102) and tender braised collard greens for a traditional Southern-style feast.

8 ounces tempeh

1 cup Good-to-Your-Gut Barbecue Sauce
(page 117)

Cut the tempeh crosswise into four equal pieces. Put in a medium saucepan, cover with water, and bring to a gentle simmer over medium-high heat. Decrease the heat to medium-low and simmer gently for 10 minutes. Drain well and pat dry. Let cool, then slice each piece crosswise into 3 or 4 slices per piece (depending on how thick you want the ribs to be), for a total of 12 to 16 slices.

Put the tempeh slices and sauce in a large bowl or on a large rimmed plate and toss gently with your hands to coat the tempeh evenly. Take care to avoid breaking the slices. Let marinate for 10 minutes.

Preheat the oven to 400 degrees F. Oil a large roasting pan (preferably nonstick) or rimmed baking sheet. Alternatively, line the pan with parchment paper or a silicone baking mat. Arrange the tempeh in a single layer in the prepared pan. Don't let the pieces touch or they won't cook properly. For extra-spicy, extra-saucy short ribs, spread the sauce remaining in the bowl evenly over each piece. Bake for 30 minutes for soft, tender short ribs, or for 40 minutes for chewier short ribs.

Barbecued Tofu Short Ribs Replace the tempeh with 12 ounces of superfirm or extra-firm tofu, well pressed (see page 28). Cut the tofu crosswise into 12 equal slices, marinate as directed, and bake for 40 minutes.

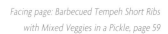

Facing page: Barbecued Tempeh Short Ribs
with Mixed Veggies in a Pickle, page 59

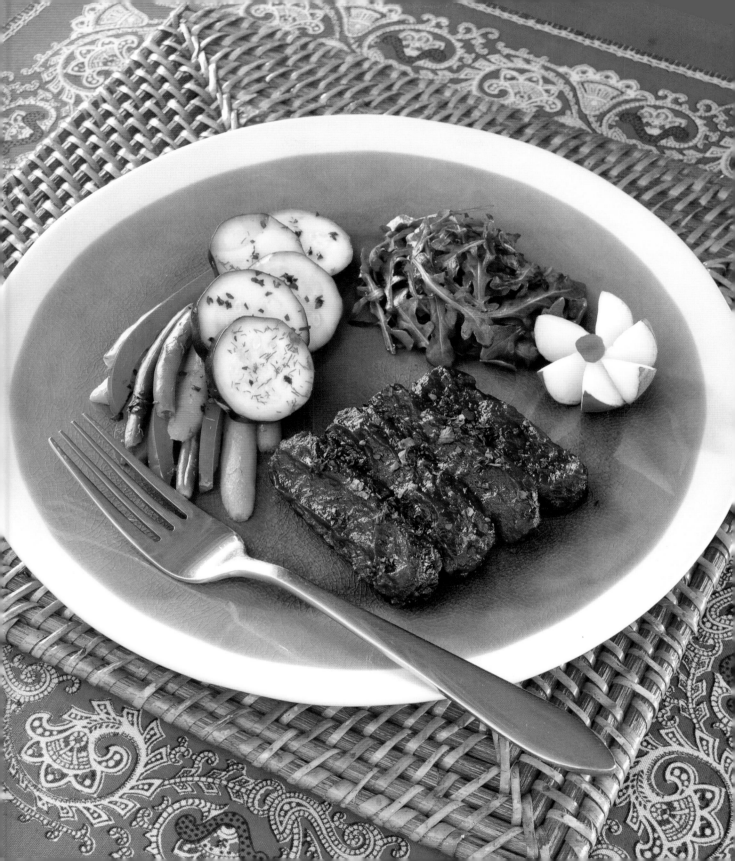

Teriyaki Tempeh

MAKES 4 SERVINGS

Per serving:

256 calories

13 g protein

16 g fat (5 g sat)

6 g carbs

956 mg sodium

105 mg calcium

1 g fiber

Tempting teriyaki tempeh pairs beautifully with hot rice and steamed broccoli, green beans, bok choy, spinach, or chard. If you or your dinner guests would appreciate a bit of extra heat, pass a small bowl of Good-to-Your-Gut Sriracha Sauce (page 56) or Mild Hot Sauce (page 54) at the table.

8 ounces tempeh

¼ cup light brown sugar, packed

¼ cup reduced-sodium tamari

¼ cup rice vinegar

1 tablespoon garlic-infused olive oil

1 tablespoon toasted sesame oil

1 teaspoon peeled and grated fresh ginger

½ teaspoon crushed red pepper flakes

1 tablespoon coconut oil

½ cup finely diced bell pepper (any color)

¼ cup scallion greens

Cut the tempeh crosswise into four equal pieces. Put in a medium saucepan, cover with water, and bring to a gentle simmer over medium-high heat. Decrease the heat to medium-low and simmer gently for 10 minutes. Drain well and pat dry. Let cool, then thinly slice each piece crosswise.

To make the sauce, put the brown sugar, tamari, vinegar, garlic-infused oil, toasted sesame oil, ginger, and red pepper flakes in a small bowl and stir or whisk until well combined.

Put the coconut oil in a large saucepan or skillet (preferably nonstick) and heat over medium heat. When hot, add bell pepper and tempeh and cook, turning frequently, until the tempeh pieces are browned on both sides, about 10 minutes. Decrease the heat to medium-low. Stir the sauce, then pour it over the tempeh. Cook, stirring gently but almost constantly, until the sauce is thickened, about 5 minutes. Sprinkle the scallion greens over the top just before serving.

Tofu, Chickpea, and Spinach Stir-Fry

A tofu-and-vegetable stir-fry makes a wholesome, light supper any day of the week. The addition of a small amount of chickpeas in this version ramps up the protein and fiber while keeping the dish low in FODMAPs. Serve it with a side of hot rice or quinoa (see table 13, page 44) or FODMAP-safe toast or crackers.

MAKES 4 SERVINGS

Per serving:
195 calories
14 g protein
9 g fat (2 g sat)
14 g carbs
54 mg sodium
210 mg calcium
5 g fiber

1 tablespoon garlic-infused olive oil

12 ounces superfirm or extra-firm tofu, pressed (see page 28) **and cut into ½-inch cubes**

¾ cup no-salt-added canned chickpeas, rinsed well and drained

1 medium orange, red, or yellow bell pepper, cut into 2-inch-long strips

1 teaspoon All-Purpose Herb Blend (page 55) **or other low-FODMAP seasoning blend**

1 teaspoon curry powder

¼ teaspoon ground turmeric

1 firm, ripe tomato, seeded and diced

¼ cup sliced scallion greens

1 cup coarsely chopped baby spinach, firmly packed

Sea salt

Freshly ground black pepper

Tabasco or Mild Hot Sauce (page 54)

Put the oil in a large skillet (preferably nonstick) and heat over medium-high heat. When hot, add the tofu, chickpeas, and bell pepper and cook, stirring frequently, until golden brown in spots, about 5 minutes. Sprinkle with the herb blend, curry powder, and turmeric and stir until evenly distributed. Decrease the heat to medium, add the tomato and scallion greens, and cook, stirring frequently, for 3 minutes. Add the spinach and stir to combine. Cover and cook until the spinach is wilted, 1 to 2 minutes. Remove from the heat and season with salt, pepper, and Tabasco to taste.

Note: Analysis doesn't include sea salt or freshly ground black pepper to taste.

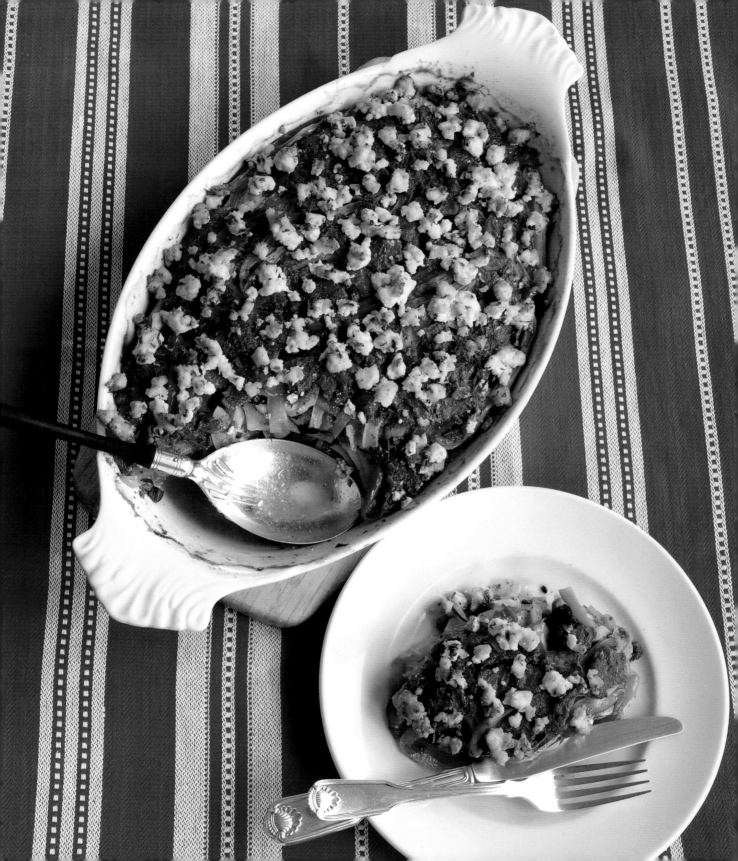

Baked Zucchini and Potatoes with Greek Tofu Feta

This hearty, low-fat casserole will fill you up without weighing you down. The long baking time infuses the flavors throughout and thoroughly tenderizes the vegetables. Serve it alone or with a large side salad for a simple but satisfying meal.

MAKES 6 SERVINGS

Per serving:
291 calories
10 g protein
11 g fat (1 g sat)
39 g carbs
540 mg sodium
190 mg calcium
8 g fiber

1 can (14.5 ounces) **no-salt-added diced tomatoes, with juice**

¼ cup minced fresh dill, or 1 tablespoon dried dill weed

2 tablespoons chopped fresh flat-leaf parsley, or 2 teaspoons dried parsley

1 tablespoon garlic-infused olive oil

½ teaspoon sea salt, plus more for sprinkling

¼ teaspoon freshly ground black pepper, plus more for sprinkling

4 medium russet potatoes, peeled and thinly sliced

2 medium or 4 small zucchini, thinly sliced on the diagonal

30 pitted kalamata or oil-cured olives, sliced or chopped

3 bell peppers (various colors), **sliced into thin strips**

1½ cups crumbled Greek Tofu Feta (page 48)

Preheat the oven to 375 degrees F. Generously oil a large roasting pan (preferably nonstick) or line it with parchment paper or a silicone baking mat.

Put the tomatoes, dill, parsley, oil, salt, and pepper in a small bowl and stir to combine.

Layer half the potatoes in the prepared roasting pan and sprinkle with salt and pepper. Top with a layer of half the zucchini, then a layer of half the olives, then a layer of half the bell peppers. Dollop half the tomato mixture over the top as evenly as possible. Layer the remaining potatoes over the tomato mixture and sprinkle them with salt and pepper. Top with a layer of the remaining zucchini, then a layer of the remaining olives, then a layer of the remaining bell peppers. Dollop the remaining tomato mixture over the top as evenly as possible. Cover with foil and bake for 1 hour and 15 minutes. Sprinkle with the feta and bake, uncovered, for 20 minutes, until the mixture is bubbly and the feta is golden brown on top. Serve hot, warm, or at room temperature.

Lemon Rice with Kale and Mint

MAKES 4 SERVINGS

Per serving:

367 calories

5 g protein

18 g fat (2 g sat)

46 g carbs

406 mg sodium

35 mg calcium

2 g fiber

With vivid, contrasting colors, this dish is a sight to behold. The aroma of mint and lemon will invigorate any sluggish appetite. This is my weekly go-to choice on days when I want something fabulous but don't feel like getting too involved in the kitchen. It's also an excellent dish for company.

2 cups water

1 cup stemmed (see box, page 96) **and finely chopped kale, packed**

1 cup white basmati or long-grain white rice

1 tablespoon lemon-infused olive oil or extra-virgin olive oil

1 tablespoon garlic-infused olive oil

1½ tablespoons dried spearmint

2 teaspoons grated lemon zest (optional)

¼ teaspoon sea salt

3 tablespoons freshly squeezed lemon juice

¼ cup thinly sliced scallion greens or chives (optional)

20 pitted kalamata or oil-cured olives, chopped or sliced

¼ cup pine nuts, raw or lightly toasted (see tip, page 111)

8 Campari or cocktail tomatoes, quartered, or 16 to 20 yellow, orange, or red grape tomatoes, halved lengthwise

Put the water and kale in a medium saucepan (preferably nonstick) and bring to a boil over medium-high heat. Decrease the heat to medium, cover, and cook until the kale is tender, 5 to 8 minutes. Add the rice, lemon-infused oil, garlic-infused oil, spearmint, optional zest, and salt and stir to combine. Decrease the heat to low, cover, and cook until the water is absorbed and the rice is tender, 15 to 18 minutes. Remove from the heat and let rest, covered, for 10 minutes. Add the lemon juice and optional scallion greens and fluff with a fork until evenly distributed. Garnish each serving with one-quarter of the olives and pine nuts. Arrange the tomatoes around the rim of each bowl with the bottom points slightly submerged beneath the rice.

Lemon Rice with Kale, Mint, and Feta Replace the olives with 1 cup of crumbled Greek Tofu Feta (page 48), or add the feta along with the olives.

Lemon Rice with Spinach, Mint, and Olives Replace the kale with 1 cup of chopped baby spinach. Add the spinach with the rice (the spinach will cook with the rice; it doesn't need to cook on its own) and proceed with the recipe as directed.

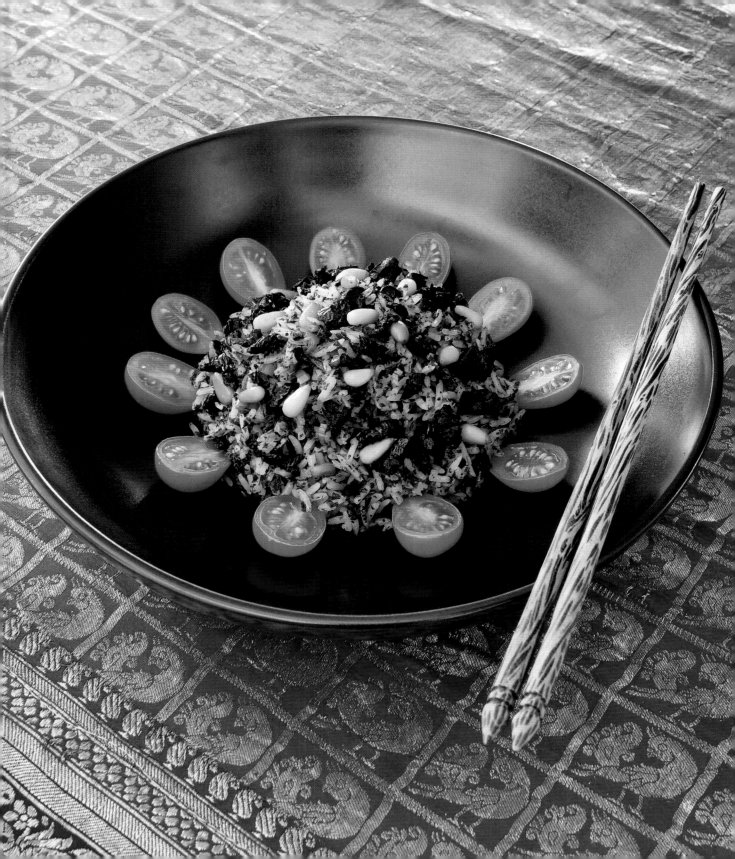

Kale, Peanut, and Pineapple Stew

MAKES 4 SERVINGS

Per serving:

489 calories

15 g protein

20 g fat (3 g sat)

61 g carbs

53 mg sodium

95 mg calcium

8 g fiber

This stew pulls together quite quickly but tastes like it cooked all day. The peanut butter mellows the large amount of Tabasco, giving the dish a surprisingly gentle bite. Serve it over your favorite low-FODMAP grain or pasta for a truly satisfying meal. The optional garnishes transform it into a company-worthy feast.

4 cups stemmed (see box) **and chopped kale, lightly packed** (about 1 large bunch**)**

⅔ cup water

1 tablespoon garlic-infused olive oil

2 cups (16 ounces) **canned crushed pineapple in juice or pineapple tidbits in juice, undrained**

½ cup no-salt-added creamy peanut butter

1 tablespoon Tabasco or Mild Hot Sauce (page 54)

Sea salt

3 cups cooked rice, quinoa, hulled millet (see table 13, page 44)**, or gluten-free pasta cooked and drained according to the package directions**

1 cup alfalfa sprouts or bean sprouts (optional)

¼ cup chopped fresh cilantro or flat-leaf parsley, lightly packed (optional)

¼ cup sliced chives or scallion greens (optional)

¼ cup chopped or crushed unsalted roasted peanuts (optional)

Put the kale, water, and oil in a large saucepan (preferably nonstick) and bring to a boil over high heat. Decrease the heat to medium-low, cover, and cook, stirring occasionally, until the kale is very tender and the water has evaporated, 15 to 20 minutes. If the water evaporates before the kale is tender, add a little more as needed. If water remains after the kale is tender, uncover, increase the heat to medium-high, and cook, stirring almost constantly, until the water evaporates. Remove from the heat.

Add the pineapple with juice and stir to combine. Add the peanut butter and Tabasco and stir until well combined. Season with salt to taste. Heat over medium heat, stirring frequently, until hot. Serve over the hot rice, garnished with the optional sprouts, cilantro, scallion greens, and/or peanuts.

Note: Analysis doesn't include sea salt to taste.

HOW TO STEM KALE, COLLARDS, AND CHARD

There are two ways to stem dark leafy greens and remove the tough inner rib. After the leaves have been thoroughly washed, fold each leaf in half with the rib facing out, then trim along the inside of the rib from top to bottom with a sharp knife. Alternatively (and this is my favorite method), hold a leaf by the end with one hand while putting the thumb and index finger of your other hand around the stem, just below the leaves. Firmly draw your fingers up along the stem, tearing off the leaves.

Ten-Minute One-Pan Pasta

This dish requires only one pan because it makes its own sauce. Once you nail the basic recipe, try adding other low-FODMAP ingredients, such as cubed firm tofu, sliced black or green olives, capers, small broccoli florets, peeled and diced eggplant, baby spinach, baby kale, sliced Swiss chard, shredded carrots, or diced or sliced bell peppers. This recipe is forgiving and flexible, so use whatever you prefer or have on hand, and have fun with it.

MAKES 4 SERVINGS

Per serving:

379 calories

7 g protein

9 g fat (1 g sat)

69 g carbs

222 mg sodium

0 mg calcium

2 g fiber

12 ounces gluten-free pasta (any shape)

12 ounces cherry or grape tomatoes, halved (or quartered if large), **or 1 can** (14.5 ounces) **no-salt-added canned tomatoes, with juice**

1 tablespoon dried basil

1 tablespoon garlic-infused olive oil

1 tablespoon basil-infused olive oil, extra-virgin olive oil, or additional garlic-infused olive oil

¼ to ½ teaspoon crushed red pepper flakes (optional)

½ teaspoon sea salt, plus more as needed

¼ teaspoon freshly ground black pepper, plus more as needed

4 cups water, plus more as needed (see tip)

¼ cup toasted pine nuts (see tip, page 111) **or vegan Parmesan cheese, for garnish**

Put the pasta, tomatoes, basil, garlic-infused oil, basil-infused oil, optional red pepper flakes, salt, pepper, and water in a deep, large saucepan or skillet. If using long noodles, such as spaghetti or linguine, the pan should be wide enough so the noodles can lay flat. Bring to a boil over high heat. Decrease the heat to medium-high and cook, stirring and turning the pasta frequently with a long-handled wooden spoon or tongs, until it is tender and the water has nearly evaporated, about 10 minutes. If the pasta is very thick or you want more sauce, add up to ½ cup of additional water during cooking. Season to taste with additional salt and pepper as desired. Garnish with the pine nuts just before serving.

One-Pan Cheesy Pasta with Veggies Omit the tomatoes and basil. Add 1½ tablespoons of freshly squeezed lemon juice, 2 teaspoons of dried chives, and ¼ teaspoon of dry mustard at the start of cooking. After the pasta has cooked for 5 minutes, stir in 1½ cups of fresh or frozen broccoli florets or cut green beans. Cover and cook, stirring frequently, until the pasta and vegetables are tender, about 5 minutes longer. Add ¼ cup of nutritional yeast flakes and stir until evenly incorporated and the sauce is smooth and creamy.

Ten-Minute One-Pan Pasta with Chickpeas Add 1 cup of canned chickpeas, rinsed well and drained, at the start of cooking.

Ten-Minute One-Pan Pasta with Tomato Purée Replace the tomatoes with 1½ cups of no-salt-added tomato purée. Decrease the water to 2½ cups and proceed with the recipe as directed.

TIP This might seem like a lot of water at the start, but it will cook off and thicken into a delicious sauce as the pasta becomes tender. If there's too much liquid at the end of the cooking time, remove the pan from the heat, cover, and let rest for 2 minutes; the pasta will absorb the excess liquid. If you prefer a saucier dish, add ½ cup of additional water at the start of cooking. Note that different types and shapes of pasta will require slightly more or less water, so adjust the amount as needed.

Eggplant and Spinach Bolognese with Pasta

MAKES 6 SERVINGS

Per serving:

332 calories

8 g protein

6 g fat (1 g sat)

63 g carbs

137 mg sodium

45 mg calcium

7 g fiber

This hearty dish comes together in under twenty minutes but tastes like it was simmering all day. The sauce is rich, thick, and spicy, and brimming with chunks of meaty eggplant. For the best results, be sure to peel the eggplant thoroughly.

12 ounces gluten-free pasta (any shape)

1 tablespoon low-FODMAP vegan butter or extra-virgin olive oil (optional)

1 tablespoon extra-virgin olive oil

1 tablespoon garlic-infused olive oil

1 eggplant (about 1 pound), **well peeled and cut into ½-inch cubes**

2 teaspoons dried basil

2 teaspoons dried oregano

½ teaspoon cayenne (optional)

¼ teaspoon sea salt, plus more as needed

4 cups no-salt-added tomato purée

4 cups chopped baby spinach, lightly packed

1 teaspoon crushed red pepper flakes (optional)

Tabasco or Mild Hot Sauce (page 54; optional)

Freshly ground black pepper

6 tablespoons raw or lightly toasted pine nuts (see tip, page 111; optional)

Cook the pasta in a large pot of boiling water according to the package directions. Drain, return to the pot or transfer to a large bowl, toss with the optional butter until it is melted and evenly distributed (this will help keep the pasta from sticking together), and cover to keep warm.

While the pasta is cooking, make the sauce. Put the extra-virgin olive oil and garlic-infused oil in a wide, large saucepan (preferably nonstick) and heat over medium-high heat. When hot, add the eggplant, basil, oregano, optional cayenne, and salt and stir until the seasonings are evenly distributed. Cook, stirring frequently, until the eggplant is soft, about 10 minutes. Add the tomato purée and bring to a simmer. Decrease the heat to medium-low and cook, stirring occasionally, for 5 minutes. Add the spinach and optional red pepper flakes and cook, stirring frequently, until the spinach is wilted and tender, about 3 minutes. Season with additional salt and Tabasco and pepper to taste. To serve, divide the pasta among six bowls. Spoon the hot sauce over the pasta and sprinkle each serving with the optional pine nuts.

Eggplant, Spinach, and Lentil Bolognese with Pasta Add 1 cup of canned lentils, rinsed well and drained, along with the tomato purée.

Zucchini and Spinach Bolognese with Pasta Replace the eggplant with 1 pound of zucchini (about 3 medium), cut into ½-inch cubes. Do not peel the zucchini.

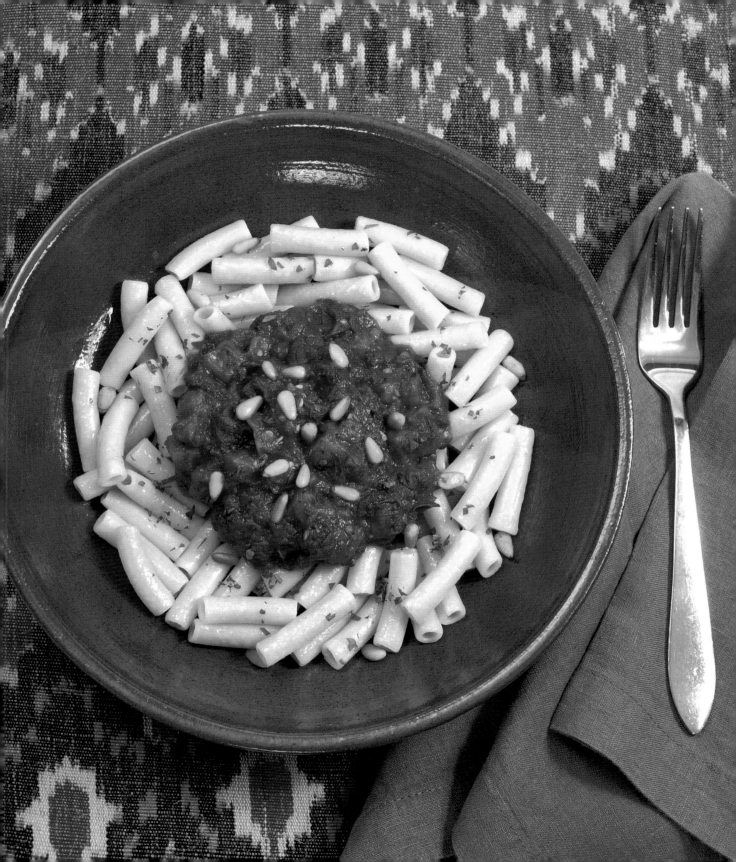

Classic Lentil Loaf

MAKES 8 SERVINGS

Per serving:

172 calories

6 g protein

11 g fat (1 g sat)

13 g carbs

370 mg sodium

35 mg calcium

2 g fiber

This scrumptious loaf belies its simplicity. It's hearty, flavorful, and great for a down-home meal or holiday gathering. Serve it with a side of mashed potatoes drizzled with Warm Nut Butter Gravy (page 108), sautéed zucchini or steamed green beans, and a salad, and you'll have yourself a low-FODMAP feast. Of course, thinly sliced leftover loaf is ideal as a sandwich filling on low-FODMAP bread spread with Good-to-Your-Gut Ketchup. If you have All-Purpose Herb Blend, Good-to-Your-Gut Ketchup, and Good-to-Your-Gut Barbecue Sauce ready-made, the loaf can be pulled together quite rapidly.

1 can (15 ounces) **no-salt-added lentils, rinsed well and drained**

1½ cups quick-cooking rolled oats

½ cup walnuts, finely chopped

¼ cup Good-to-Your-Gut Ketchup (page 57), **plus more for garnish**

¼ cup Good-to-Your-Gut Barbecue Sauce (page 117)

4 tablespoons no-salt-added creamy peanut butter

2 tablespoons Dijon or spicy brown mustard

2 tablespoons reduced-sodium tamari

1 tablespoon All-Purpose Herb Blend (page 55)

1 tablespoon garlic-infused olive oil

Preheat the oven to 350 degrees F. Oil an 8-inch square baking pan.

Put all the ingredients in a large bowl and stir until well combined. Transfer to the oiled baking pan and pack the mixture down firmly and evenly. Bake for 45 to 50 minutes, until firm, golden brown, and a little crusty on top. Let rest for 10 minutes before slicing and serving. Garnish with additional ketchup as desired before or after slicing.

Loaded Baked Potatoes

Baked spuds are a trusty comfort food, and they're especially soothing to a gut in turmoil when not much else seems appetizing. They also make a fabulous foundation for a simple yet satisfying main dish when topped with a creamy sauce or hearty protein. Some people struggle with nailing the perfect baked potato, so this recipe removes all the guesswork. If you have difficulty digesting too much fiber, skip the skins. The potato flesh is low in calories and rich in potassium, magnesium, iron, and vitamin C. Not too shabby!

MAKES 2 SERVINGS

See photo, page 103

POTATOES

2 russet potatoes

Olive oil (optional)

TOPPING SELECTIONS (choose one or two)

Any sauce or dressing from Getting Sauced (pages 108 to 118)

Barbecued Tempeh Short Ribs (page 88)

Barbecued Tofu Short Ribs (page 88)

Chickenless Chicken Salad (page 52)

Chive Cheese Spread (page 60)

Curried Walnut Pâté (page 62)

Dilled Lemon-Caper Sauce (page 82)

Ginger-Glazed Tempeh Filets (page 87)

Greek Tofu Feta (page 48)

Green Bean and Walnut Pâté (page 62)

Herbed Tempeh Nuggets (page 51)

I Can't Believe It's Not Cheese Sauce (page 60)

I Can't Believe It's Not Cheese Spread (page 60)

Lentil and Walnut Pâté (page 62)

Lentil Hummus (page 61)

Lentil Salad with Chard and Tomatoes (page 130)

Lentil-Chickpea Hummus (page 61)

Maple-Miso Tofu (page 50)

Orange Cheese Spread (page 60)

Pecan Pâté (page 62)

Remoulade Sauce (page 84)

Seitan strips

Sriracha Mayo (page 56)

Sriracha-Mustard Mayo (page 56)

Teriyaki Tempeh (page 90)

Two-Way Tempeh Salad (page 127)

Vegan butter, low-FODMAP

Vegan cheese

Vegan mayonnaise

Walnut Pâté (page 62)

Zucchini Hummus (page 61)

VEGGIES (choose one or more)

Alfalfa sprouts	**Mesclun**
Baby arugula	**Pitted olives, sliced**
Baby kale	**Radishes, sliced or diced**
Baby spinach	**Romaine, shredded**
Bean sprouts	**Scallion greens, sliced**
Bell pepper (any color), **diced**	**Tomato, seeded and chopped**
Carrot, shredded	**Water chestnuts, sliced or diced**
Chives, sliced	**Yellow squash, diced or shredded**
English or mini cucumber, sliced or diced	**Zucchini, diced or shredded**

Preheat the oven to 350 degrees F. Scrub the potatoes with a stiff brush under cold running water. Pat dry. Using a standard table fork, deeply pierce each potato all over in eight to ten places. The fork should enter the flesh a bit and not just break the surface of the skin.

For a more tender and flavorful skin, put the potatoes on a paper towel or in a bowl and lightly coat them all over with a small amount of oil, rubbing the oil in with your hands.

To keep the oven rack clean and catch any drippings, put a sheet of parchment paper or a silicone baking mat on the center rack of the oven and put the potatoes on it. Bake for 60 to 75 minutes, until a fork slides easily into the flesh. (The baking time needed will depend on the age, size, and moisture content of the potatoes.) Remove from the oven and let rest for 10 minutes before serving. (Note: If you're baking more than two potatoes, extend the cooking time by 5 minutes for each additional potato.)

To serve, create a dotted line from end to end of each potato using the tines of a table fork. Crack open the potato by gently squeezing the ends toward each other. The potato will pop open (take care, as it will emit some steam). Gently push the flesh up from the bottom and fluff with the fork. Serve hot, loaded with the toppings and veggies of your choice.

Facing page: Loaded Baked Potatoes (page 101),
in back, topped with Lentil Salad with Chard and Tomatoes (page 130) and Greek Tofu Feta (page 48),
in front, with Yum-Yum Sauce (page 108) and veggies

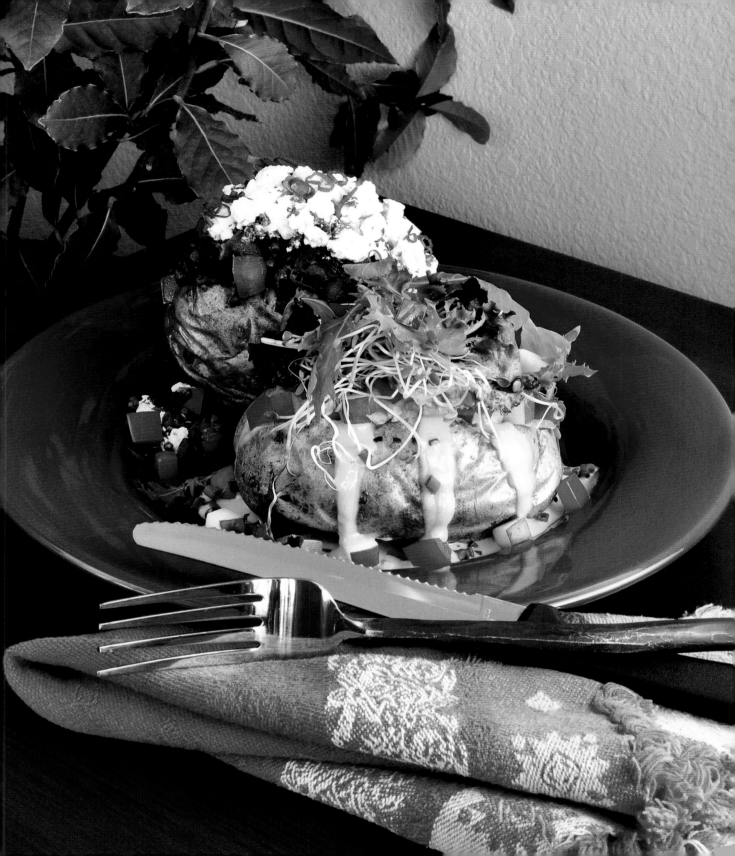

Bliss Bowls

MAKES AS MANY SERVINGS
AS YOU LIKE

You could probably serve Bliss Bowls every night of the week and never repeat the same one twice. These blissful bowls of cooked grain, low-FODMAP vegan protein, and raw and cooked veggies can be topped with whatever low-FODMAP sauce or seasoning strikes your fancy. They're perfect for everyday fare or even to serve to guests. Plus, they're a great way to use up leftover veggies, sauces, and dressings. When you don't know what to make for dinner, make it a Bliss Bowls night!

Step 1 Prepare the grain or starch. Cook enough rice, quinoa, hulled millet, or polenta for each person to have at least ½ to ⅔ cup of cooked grain (see table 13, page 44). Put the water in a medium saucepan (preferably nonstick), add ¼ teaspoon of salt per cup of grain if desired, and bring to a boil over medium-high heat. Add the grain, stir, cover, and decrease the heat to low. Let millet, quinoa, rice, and wild rice cook undisturbed. When cooking polenta, stir occasionally with a long-handled spoon. Polenta will sputter vigorously and splatter, so stand back to prevent getting burned when you lift the lid and stir.

When the grain is finished cooking, remove from the heat and let rest, covered, for 10 minutes. For pilaf, fluff with a fork before serving. For polenta, stir vigorously with a wooden spoon until creamy before serving.

As an alternative to grain or polenta, use gluten-free pasta cooked in boiling water according to the package directions, or try steamed, roasted, or mashed potatoes.

Step 2 Choose a protein. The following are some tasty low-FODMAP selections:

Barbecued Tempeh Short Ribs (page 88)

Barbecued Tofu Short Ribs (page 88)

Breakfast Scramble (page 78)

Chickenless Chicken (page 52), **sliced into very thin strips**

Chickpeas, canned, rinsed and drained (no more than ¼ cup per serving)

Chive Cheese Spread (page 60)

Ginger-Glazed Tempeh Filets (page 87)

Herbed Tempeh Nuggets (page 51)

I Can't Believe It's Not Cheese Spread (page 60)

Lemon-Pepper Tofu (page 50)

Lentil Hummus (page 61)

Lentil-Chickpea Hummus (page 61)

Lentils, canned, rinsed and drained (no more than ½ cup per serving)

Maple-Miso Tofu (page 50)

Pecan Pâté (page 62)

Seitan strips or cubes

Tempeh Bacon (page 49)

Teriyaki Tempeh (page 90)

Tofu Bacon Strips or Slabs (page 49)

Tofu, Chickpea, and Spinach Stir-Fry (page 91)

Two-Way Tempeh Salad (page 127)

Walnut and Green Bean Pâté (page 62)

Walnut and Lentil Pâté (page 62)

Walnut Pâté (page 62)

Zucchini Hummus (page 61)

Step 3 Pick your veggies. Vegetables can be either raw or cooked (steamed, roasted, or stir-fried). For a list of choices, see page 37, or try roasted vegetables (page 82). If you put raw baby spinach or baby kale under the hot grain, the greens will wilt slightly, creating a pleasing, soft texture. Tougher or firmer vegetables, such as diced or shredded carrots, chopped mature kale, or chopped collard greens, can be cooked along with the grain: simply put the veggies in the saucepan with the water and grain before covering with the lid. Other raw or cooked veggies can be put on the bottom of the bowl, mixed in with the hot grain, scattered over the top (either under or over the protein), or arranged in individual piles around the grain at the edges of the bowl. Tender raw veggies, such as salad greens, baby lettuces, baby arugula, alfalfa or bean sprouts, and tomatoes, are best piled on top or arranged around the edges to avoid getting crushed or bruised.

Step 4 Select a sauce and/or seasonings. Sauces, condiments, and garnishes will tie everything together. Choose any of the recipes in the Getting Sauced chapter (pages 108 to 118) or try Dilled Lemon-Caper Sauce (page 82), Remoulade Sauce (page 84), or Sriracha Dressing, Sriracha Mayo, or Sriracha-Mustard Mayo (page 56). You can also add pickles or relish (page 59), fresh herbs, Tabasco or Mild Hot Sauce (page 54), plain vegan mayonnaise, spicy mayo (vegan mayonnaise with a little Tabasco, or Mild Hot Sauce or Mild Hot Chile Paste, page 54, mixed in), tamari, toasted sesame oil, extra-virgin olive oil, basil- or herb-infused olive oil, garlic-infused olive oil, lemon-infused olive oil, freshly squeezed lemon or lime juice, rice vinegar, or balsamic vinegar in addition to or instead of a sauce.

Step 5 Assemble the bowls. Put any veggies you'd like to soften on the bottom of the bowl. Top with the hot cooked grain, raw or cooked veggies, and a protein option, and end with tender lettuces or other tender vegetables (sprouts, baby arugula, and/or tomatoes) or vegetable garnishes. Alternatively, put the grain in the center of the bowl or off to one side and arrange the protein option and vegetables individually in small piles around it. Top with your choice of sauce or seasonings and/or sprinkle with Seasoned Pumpkin or Sunflower Seeds (page 53) or raw or toasted nuts or seeds (see variation, page 53).

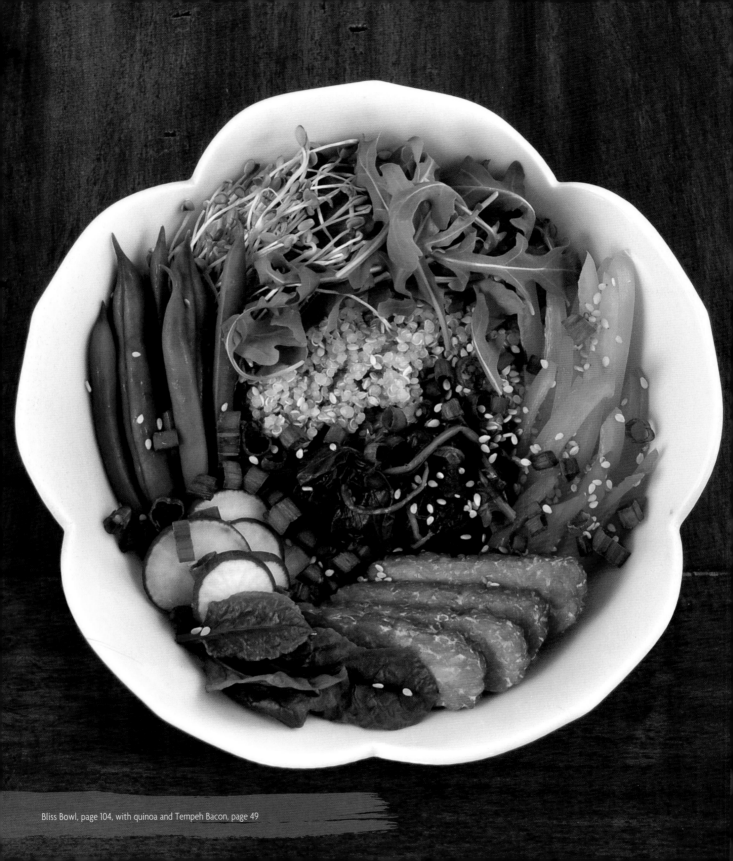

Bliss Bowl, page 104, with quinoa and Tempeh Bacon, page 49

9

Getting Sauced

Yum-Yum Sauce

**MAKES 1⅓ CUPS,
6 SERVINGS**

Per serving:

141 calories

3 g protein

12 g fat (2 g sat)

6 g carbs

75 mg sodium

12 mg calcium

2 g fiber

This sauce is a high-protein, low-FODMAP dream come true. It's rich and creamy and bursting with flavor, which makes it a fantastic go-to sauce to top Bliss Bowls (page 104), gluten-free pasta, Loaded Baked Potatoes (page 101), baked tofu or tempeh, or any low-FODMAP grain. Because it contains just a small amount of chickpeas, the protein content is given a boost while the FODMAPs remain in the safe range.

½ cup no-salt-added canned chickpeas, rinsed well and drained

¼ cup water

¼ cup freshly squeezed lemon juice

3 tablespoons extra-virgin olive oil

2 tablespoons nutritional yeast flakes

2 tablespoons no-salt-added peanut butter, almond butter, or tahini

1 tablespoon garlic-infused olive oil

¾ teaspoon curry powder

½ teaspoon dried cilantro

½ teaspoon dried oregano

¼ teaspoon sea salt

Put all the ingredients in a blender and process on high speed until the chickpeas are thoroughly pulverized and the sauce is completely smooth. Transfer to a storage container and refrigerate for 12 to 24 hours before serving to let the flavors meld. Store in a sealed container in the refrigerator.

Warm Nut Butter Gravy

**MAKES 1¾ CUPS,
6 SERVINGS**

Per serving:

152 calories

6 g protein

12 g fat (1 g sat)

8 g carbs

341 mg sodium

40 mg calcium

1 g fiber

This effortless sauce is quite luscious and can be used in place of white sauce in most conventional recipes or used as a gravy spooned over baked tempeh or tofu, mashed or baked potatoes (see page 102), or rice-and-veggie bowls.

4 tablespoons no-salt-added creamy peanut butter

4 tablespoons almond butter, tahini, or additional peanut butter

4 tablespoons chickpea or light miso

2 tablespoons freshly squeezed lemon juice

¾ cup hot water, as needed

Put the peanut butter, almond butter, miso, and lemon juice in a small bowl and stir well to make a thick paste. Gradually stir or whisk in the water, using just enough to achieve the desired consistency; beat vigorously after each addition until smooth and creamy. Alternatively, put all the ingredients in a blender and process until smooth.

Serve immediately or, to warm the gravy further, transfer to a small saucepan (preferably nonstick) and briefly heat over medium-low heat, stirring frequently, for about 1 minute. Do not boil. If the gravy thickens too much, whisk in a small amount of additional water, 1 teaspoon at a time, until the desired consistency is achieved.

Gingered Nut Butter Gravy Omit the lemon juice and add 2 teaspoons of peeled and grated fresh ginger and a pinch of cayenne. Add more water as needed to achieve the desired consistency.

TIP Store leftovers in a sealed container in the refrigerator. To serve, warm per the instructions above.

Good-to-Your-Gut Roasted-Tomato Salsa

Bring on the corn chips! Whether you're by yourself or surrounded by friends, when you serve this unique low-FODMAP salsa, there's going to be a party.

1 can (14 to 15 ounces) **no-salt-added fire-roasted diced tomatoes, drained**

1 red bell pepper, diced

¼ cup sliced scallion greens

¼ cup chopped fresh cilantro or flat-leaf parsley, packed

2 tablespoons freshly squeezed lime juice

1 jalapeño chile, seeded and diced (optional)

1 teaspoon ground cumin (optional)

Sea salt

Freshly ground black pepper

Tabasco or Mild Hot Sauce (page 54)

MAKES 1½ CUPS,
6 SERVINGS

Per serving:
26 calories
1 g protein
0 g fat (0 g sat)
5 g carbs
10 mg sodium
65 mg calcium
2 g fiber

Put the tomatoes, bell pepper, scallion greens, cilantro, lime juice, optional chile, and optional cumin in a medium bowl and stir until well combined. Season with salt, pepper, and Tabasco to taste. Store in a covered container in the refrigerator.

Pineapple Party Salsa Add 1 cup of chopped fresh, defrosted frozen, or canned pineapple (packed in juice), well drained.

Note: Analysis doesn't include sea salt, freshly ground black pepper, or Tabasco to taste.

Spicy Peanut Sauce

**MAKES 1 1/3 CUPS,
5 SERVINGS**

Per serving:
186 calories
6 g protein
14 g fat (2 g sat)
6 g carbs
300 mg sodium
9 mg calcium
2 g fiber

This delectable sauce is always a big hit with people of all ages. Serve it over gluten-free pasta, low-FODMAP grains, baked potatoes (see page 102), steamed vegetables, or even salad greens. It's exceedingly flavorful, so a little goes a long way.

½ cup no-salt-added creamy peanut butter

2 tablespoons reduced-sodium tamari

1 teaspoon garlic-infused olive oil

1 teaspoon rice vinegar, plus more as needed

1 teaspoon pure maple syrup or unbleached cane sugar

½ teaspoon ground ginger

⅔ cup water, as needed

Thai Red Curry Paste, Mild Hot Sauce, Mild Hot Chile Paste (page 54), **Tabasco, or cayenne**

2 tablespoons thinly sliced scallion greens or chives, or 2 teaspoons dried chives (optional)

Put the peanut butter in a small bowl. Stir in the tamari, oil, vinegar, maple syrup, and ginger, beating vigorously with a wooden spoon. Gradually beat in half the water, then whisk in just enough additional water to achieve the desired consistency. Alternatively, put the ingredients in a blender and process until smooth. Season with curry paste and additional rice vinegar to taste. Stir in the optional scallion greens. Store in a covered container in the refrigerator. The sauce will thicken a bit when chilled and might separate a little. Stir well and add a small amount of water before using if necessary.

TIP The sauce may be warmed in a small saucepan over low heat if desired. The sauce will thicken when heated, so add more water as needed.

Note: Analysis doesn't include Thai Red Curry Paste to taste.

Red Pepper and Pine Nut Sauce

This sauce can't be beat for its exquisite flavor and versatility. It's sensational on vegetables, gluten-free pasta, Loaded Baked Potatoes (page 101), low-FODMAP grains, and Bliss Bowls (page 104). It's so scrummy you'll be tempted to stick your face in the blender and lick it clean, but for safety's sake, please use a spatula.

**MAKES 1¼ CUPS,
5 SERVINGS**

Per serving:
109 calories
2 g protein
11 g fat (1 g sat)
3 g carbs
236 mg sodium
1 mg calcium
1 g fiber

1 cup roasted red bell peppers (about 2 peppers), **rinsed well and drained** (see recipe, page 57)

2 tablespoons extra-virgin olive oil

2 tablespoons pine nuts, lightly toasted (see tip) **and cooled**

1 tablespoon balsamic vinegar

1 tablespoon garlic-infused olive oil

1 teaspoon dried basil

½ teaspoon sea salt

Pinch ground allspice

Remove and discard any blackened skin from the peppers. Split open the peppers and remove and discard any seeds clinging to the interior or ribs. Put the peppers and all the other ingredients in a blender and process until smooth. Store in a covered container in the refrigerator.

TIP To toast pine nuts, put the nuts in a small skillet (preferably nonstick) and heat over medium-high heat. Cook, stirring constantly, until golden brown and fragrant, about 3 minutes. Immediately transfer to a plate (otherwise, the nuts will stick to the skillet and burn) and let cool.

Fresh Basil Pesto

MAKES ½ CUP, 4 SERVINGS

Per serving:

125 calories

2 g protein

12 g fat (1 g sat)

3 g carbs

170 mg sodium

9 mg calcium

1 g fiber

Wondering what to do with all the basil overtaking your garden? Here's the perfect solution. Pesto made with fresh basil dramatically boosts the flavor of anything it touches. Spoon it over gluten-free pasta, spaghetti squash, potatoes, rice, or veggies. Or try it as a spread inside a low-FODMAP vegan grilled cheese sandwich. Pure heaven!

1 cup fresh basil leaves, firmly packed

⅓ cup walnuts or pine nuts

1½ tablespoons chickpea or light miso

1 tablespoon extra-virgin olive oil

1 tablespoon garlic-infused olive oil

¼ teaspoon sea salt (optional)

Put all the ingredients in a food processor (for a pesto with more texture) or high-speed blender (for a smoother pesto) and process until smooth. Serve immediately.

Arugula-Spinach Pesto Replace the basil with ½ cup of baby arugula, firmly packed, and ½ cup of baby spinach, firmly packed.

Cilantro Pesto Replace the basil with 1 cup of stemmed fresh cilantro leaves, firmly packed.

Kale Pesto Replace the basil with 2 cups of stemmed (see box, page 96) and firmly packed kale. Steam the kale until very tender, about 10 minutes. Let cool. Squeeze out the moisture with your hands and coarsely chop. You should have about 1 cup of cooked leaves. Put in a food processor or high-speed blender with the remaining ingredients and process until smooth.

Herbed Balsamic Dressing

MAKES ½ CUP, 4 SERVINGS

Per serving:

82 calories

0 g protein

7 g fat (1 g sat)

4 g carbs

116 mg sodium

8 mg calcium

0 g fiber

This low-FODMAP dressing rivals any store-bought variety. It's a breeze to make, even at the last minute, because it uses staples you likely already have in your pantry. Although it's delightful drizzled over green salads and sliced fresh tomatoes, it's equally delicious on grains or Bliss Bowls (page 104). Purchase the highest-quality balsamic vinegar you can find (see Resources, page 133). True aged balsamics are richer, thicker, and more flavorful than cheaper versions. Although they're more expensive, you get what you pay for. The trade-off is that you don't need to use as much and the taste will be incomparable.

1 tablespoon extra-virgin olive oil

1 tablespoon garlic-infused olive oil

½ teaspoon liquid sunflower lecithin
(see box, page 114; optional)

6 tablespoons balsamic vinegar

1 teaspoon dried chives

½ teaspoon dried basil

½ teaspoon dried oregano

½ teaspoon dried parsley

¼ teaspoon sea salt

¼ teaspoon freshly ground black pepper

Put the olive oil, garlic-infused oil, and optional lecithin in a small bowl or measuring cup and whisk until completely emulsified. Put the vinegar, chives, basil, oregano, parsley, salt, and pepper in a separate small bowl and whisk to combine. Gradually whisk the oil mixture into the vinegar mixture, pouring it in a slow, thin stream and whisking vigorously after each addition until well combined and emulsified. Pour into a small glass jar and seal tightly. Shake well before using.

Thai Hot-and-Sour Dressing

This dressing is phenomenal on Bliss Bowls (page 104), stir-fried vegetables, or gluten-free grains. For a quick and fabulous pad thai, toss it with wide rice noodles or rice linguine, crumbled firm tofu, chopped fresh cilantro, shredded carrots, thinly sliced scallion greens, fresh bean sprouts, and chopped roasted peanuts.

MAKES ⅔ CUP, 4 SERVINGS

Per serving:
132 calories
4 g protein
10 g fat (1 g sat)
6 g carbs
355 mg sodium
10 mg calcium
1 g fiber

¼ cup freshly squeezed lime juice

3 tablespoons no-salt-added creamy or crunchy peanut butter

2 tablespoons reduced-sodium tamari

1 tablespoon toasted sesame oil

1 tablespoon unbleached cane sugar

1 teaspoon dried basil

1 teaspoon garlic-infused olive oil

½ teaspoon ground ginger

½ teaspoon dried spearmint

¼ teaspoon crushed red pepper flakes

¼ teaspoon Thai Red Curry Paste (page 54), Mild Hot Sauce (page 54), or Tabasco, plus more as needed (optional)

Put all the ingredients in a small bowl and whisk vigorously until smooth and well combined. Add more chile paste to taste if desired. Pour into a small glass jar and seal tightly. Store at room temperature. Shake well before using.

Pennsylvania Dutch Sweet-and-Sour Dressing

MAKES 1 CUP, 8 SERVINGS

Per serving:

131 calories

0 g protein

14 g fat (2 g sat)

3 g carbs

55 mg sodium

0 mg calcium

0 g fiber

Sweet-and-sour dressings typically contain onion, but with garlic-infused oil, you can effortlessly replicate the tantalizing sweet-and-sour flavor without upsetting your sensitive digestive system. This dressing is so good you'll want to pour it over more than just salad. It's ideal for marinating warm steamed veggies, especially kale, cabbage, or cut green beans, and it's a classic tossed with raw baby spinach and Tempeh Bacon (page 49).

6 tablespoons extra-virgin olive oil

2 tablespoons garlic-infused olive oil

½ teaspoon liquid sunflower lecithin (see box, below; optional)

¼ cup unbleached cane sugar

¼ cup cider vinegar

½ teaspoon dry mustard

½ teaspoon paprika

¼ teaspoon whole celery seeds, or ⅛ teaspoon ground celery seeds (optional)

¼ teaspoon sea salt

Put the extra-virgin olive oil, garlic-infused oil, and optional lecithin in a small bowl or measuring cup and whisk until completely emulsified. Put the sugar, vinegar, dry mustard, paprika, optional celery seeds, and salt in a separate small bowl and whisk to combine. Gradually whisk the oil mixture into the vinegar mixture, pouring it in a slow, thin stream and whisking vigorously after each addition until well combined and emulsified. Pour into a small glass jar and seal tightly. Store at room temperature. Shake well before using.

THE SUNNY SIDE OF LECITHIN

Lecithin, a yellow-brown fatty substance found naturally in egg yolks, soybeans, and sunflower seeds, is a necessary component of every cell in the human body. Recently, lecithin has been elevated to the status of superfood because of numerous health benefits attributed to it, from aiding in the treatment of neurological and cardiovascular diseases to improving digestion, brain health, and memory. Unlike soy lecithin, which is chemically extracted, sunflower lecithin is typically cold-pressed from the seed, using the same type of extraction process as extra-virgin olive oil.

Lecithin is used in the food industry to add a creamy texture to a broad variety of items, including almond milk, chocolate, vegan butter, and various baked goods. In salad dressings, it works as a natural thickener, stabilizer, and emulsifier that helps keep the oil from separating out. It also makes dressings creamier and more luxurious. Although lecithin is available in granular or liquid form, the liquid will work best in homemade salad dressings. It's very sticky, so oil your measuring spoon first and the lecithin will slide right off. Look for liquid sunflower lecithin at natural food stores in the supplement aisle or online. If you choose to not include the lecithin, the dressing won't be quite as thick and creamy, but it will still be delicious.

Lemon-Tahini Dressing

This dressing is a bit of a chameleon. By cutting higher-FODMAP tahini with lower-FODMAP peanut butter, you can indulge in a larger portion while experiencing full tahini flavor and keeping the FODMAPs under control. Bound to become a staple in your repertoire, this reliable favorite is creamy and thick with a tart, lemony edge. Spoon it over salads, Bliss Bowls (page 104), Tortilla Pull-Aparts (page 84), grains, or veggies.

MAKES 1 ⅓ CUPS, 4 SERVINGS

Per serving:
218 calories
6 g protein
18 g fat (3 g sat)
7 g carbs
127 mg sodium
62 mg calcium
3 g fiber

4 tablespoons tahini

4 tablespoons no-salt-added creamy peanut butter

½ cup water, plus more as needed

3 tablespoons freshly squeezed lemon juice, plus more as needed

2 teaspoons garlic-infused olive oil

¼ teaspoon sea salt, plus more as needed

Cayenne (optional)

Put the tahini and peanut butter in a small bowl. Gradually whisk in the water, beating vigorously after each addition, until smooth and creamy. Whisk in the lemon juice and oil, beating vigorously until smooth and well incorporated. Whisk in the salt and season with cayenne to taste if desired. If the dressing is too thick, add more water, 1 teaspoon at a time, until the desired consistency is achieved. Add more lemon juice or salt to taste. Alternatively, put the ingredients in a blender and process until smooth. Store in a covered container in the refrigerator. The dressing will thicken a bit when chilled. Stir well and add a small amount of water before using if necessary.

Chive-Tahini Dressing Whisk in 2 tablespoons of dried chives along with the salt and cayenne.

Lemon-Tahini Spread Decrease the water to ⅓ cup. Use as a spread for sandwiches (using 100% sourdough spelt or wheat bread or gluten-free vegan bread) or low-FODMAP vegan crackers, or as a dip for low-FODMAP veggies.

TIP The consistency of tahini and peanut butter can vary greatly, from runny to superthick. Increase or decrease the amount of water in this recipe accordingly.

Classic Vinaigrette and Marinade

**MAKES ⅔ CUP,
6 SERVINGS**

Per serving:

162 calories

0 g protein

19 g fat (3 g sat)

0 g carbs

167 mg sodium

0 mg calcium

0 g fiber

This is an excellent staple to count on whenever you need a salad dressing or marinade that everyone is sure to love. It's rich, but because it's so flavorful, a little is all you'll need to make your dishes pop. Use it to dress plain or fancy salads or coleslaw, or try it as a marinade for firm tofu or tempeh.

7 tablespoons extra-virgin olive oil

1 tablespoon garlic-infused olive oil

½ teaspoon liquid sunflower lecithin
(see box, page 114; optional)

2 tablespoons champagne vinegar or white wine vinegar

1 tablespoon freshly squeezed lemon juice

1 teaspoon Dijon or spicy brown mustard

½ teaspoon sea salt

¼ teaspoon freshly ground black pepper

¼ teaspoon unbleached cane sugar

Put the olive oil, garlic-infused oil, and optional lecithin in a small bowl or measuring cup and whisk until completely emulsified. Put the vinegar, lemon juice, mustard, salt, pepper, and sugar in a separate small bowl and whisk to combine. Gradually whisk the oil mixture into the vinegar mixture, pouring it in a slow, thin stream and whisking vigorously after each addition until well combined and emulsified. Alternatively, put all the ingredients in a blender and process until smooth and emulsified. Pour into a small glass jar and seal tightly. Store at room temperature. Shake well before using.

Basic Creamy Dressing After whisking the oil mixture into the vinegar mixture, whisk in 3 to 5 tablespoons of vegan mayonnaise until completely smooth. Whisk vigorously or process in a blender for the smoothest results. Season with additional lemon juice, salt, and pepper to taste. Store in the refrigerator. May be combined with any of the other variations that follow.

Greek Lemon Vinaigrette Omit the vinegar and mustard. Increase the lemon juice to 3 tablespoons and add 1 teaspoon of dried oregano to the vinegar mixture.

Herb Vinaigrette Add 1 teaspoon of All-Purpose Herb Blend (page 55) and 1 teaspoon of dried chives to the vinegar mixture.

Italian Vinaigrette Omit the mustard. Replace the champagne vinegar with red wine vinegar and add 1 teaspoon of dried basil, 1 teaspoon of dried oregano, and a pinch of crushed red pepper flakes to the vinegar mixture.

Noochy Dressing Omit the salt. Add 2 tablespoons of nutritional yeast flakes and 1 tablespoon of reduced-sodium tamari to the vinegar mixture. Put all the ingredients in a blender and process until smooth, thick, and emulsified.

Poppy Seed Dressing Omit the pepper. Add 3 tablespoons of additional sugar and 2 teaspoons of black poppy seeds to the vinegar mixture.

Good-to-Your-Gut Barbecue Sauce

Hot, smoky, sweet, and tangy low-FODMAP barbecue sauce has arrived! Add a spoonful to Bliss Bowls (page 104), Breakfast Scramble (page 78), baked potatoes (see page 102), or roasted veggies (page 82) and instantly pump up the flavor. This sauce packs quite a potent kick, so if your tummy prefers a milder version, try the variation that follows.

MAKES 1 CUP, 4 SERVINGS

Per serving:
52 calories
2 g protein
0 g fat (0 g sat)
12 g carbs
194 mg sodium
7 mg calcium
1 g fiber

1 cup no-salt-added tomato purée

5 tablespoons light brown sugar

3 tablespoons red wine vinegar

1 tablespoon reduced-sodium tamari

1½ teaspoons paprika

½ teaspoon dry mustard

½ teaspoon freshly ground black pepper

⅛ teaspoon smoked paprika, or 2 drops liquid smoke

⅛ teaspoon cayenne

⅛ teaspoon Tabasco or Mild Hot Sauce (page 54)

Put all the ingredients in a deep, medium saucepan (preferably nonstick) and whisk until well combined. Bring to a simmer over medium-high heat. Decrease the heat to medium-low, partially cover to minimize splatters, and simmer, stirring occasionally, until reduced and thickened, 30 to 40 minutes. Adjust the heat as necessary to maintain a simmer, and stir more frequently toward the end when the sauce has begun to thicken. Stand back when lifting the lid and stirring to avoid getting splattered or burned. Let cool completely before storing. Store in a covered container in the refrigerator.

Good-to-Your-Gut Mild Barbecue Sauce Decrease the dry mustard to ¼ teaspoon, decrease the black pepper to ¼ teaspoon, and omit the cayenne and Tabasco.

Good-to-Your-Gut Marinara Sauce

**MAKES 2 CUPS,
4 SERVINGS**

Per serving:

121 calories

3 g protein

5 g fat (1 g sat)

15 g carbs

265 mg sodium

6 mg calcium

3 g fiber

It's almost impossible to find bottled marinara sauce without onion or garlic, but it's quite easy to make a fast and flavorful low-FODMAP version at home. This is a splendid marinara sauce you can use on pasta, polenta (see table 13, page 44), baked potatoes (see page 102), or Bliss Bowls (page 104).

3 cups no-salt-added tomato purée

1½ tablespoons garlic-infused olive oil

1 teaspoon dried basil, crushed between your fingers

½ teaspoon dried oregano, crushed between your fingers

½ teaspoon sea salt

½ teaspoon freshly ground black pepper

¼ teaspoon crushed red pepper flakes (optional)

Put all the ingredients in a deep, large saucepan (preferably nonstick) and stir to combine. Bring to a simmer over medium-high heat. Decrease the heat to medium-low, partially cover to minimize splatters, and simmer, stirring occasionally, until reduced and slightly thickened, 35 to 40 minutes. Adjust the heat as necessary to maintain a simmer, and stir more frequently toward the end when the sauce has begun to thicken. Stand back when lifting the lid and stirring to avoid getting splattered or burned. Let cool completely before storing. Store in a covered container in the refrigerator.

Lentil Bolognese Sauce Add 1 cup of canned lentils, rinsed well and drained, before cooking. Add more basil, oregano, salt, pepper, and red pepper flakes to taste.

Puttanesca Sauce Add ½ cup of chopped black olives and 2 tablespoons of drained capers to the sauce before cooking.

10

Soup, Sandwich, and Salad Bar

Creamy Vegetable Soup

This thick, rich, creamy soup is very easy to make, highly nutritious, and so soothing on days when a tender tummy is aching for comfort food. It also allows for plenty of creativity and variations, so feel free to use whatever favorite low-FODMAP veggies you have on hand. Leftovers store well in the refrigerator. Just reheat them carefully so the soup doesn't curdle or burn.

6 tablespoons no-salt-added creamy peanut butter

2 tablespoons chickpea or light miso

2 tablespoons reduced-sodium tamari

1 tablespoon garlic-infused olive oil

5½ cups water or Good-to-Your-Gut Vegetable Stock (page 58)

6 tablespoons white basmati rice

2 teaspoons peeled and grated fresh ginger

1 cup diced carrots

1 cup stemmed (see box, page 96) **and chopped kale, firmly packed**

1 cup diced zucchini

½ teaspoon freshly ground black pepper

TIP For an even richer, thicker soup, stir in 2 tablespoons of tahini, almond butter, or additional peanut butter along with the peanut butter mixture.

Put the peanut butter, miso, tamari, and oil in a small bowl and stir to form a smooth, thick paste. Gradually add ½ cup of the water, stirring vigorously until smooth and creamy.

Put the remaining 5 cups of water in a large soup pot (preferably nonstick). Add the rice and ginger and stir to combine. Add the carrots and kale and bring to a boil over medium-high heat. Decrease the heat to medium-low, cover, and cook, stirring occasionally, until the kale is tender, 15 to 18 minutes. Adjust the heat as necessary to maintain a gentle simmer. Add the zucchini, cover, and cook until all the vegetables and the rice are very tender, 3 to 5 minutes.

Gradually stir the peanut butter mixture into the soup, stirring constantly and mixing well until the soup is creamy. Stir in the pepper. Do not boil.

Variations

- Replace the kale with 1 cup of fresh or frozen cut green beans, in 1-inch pieces.
- Replace the kale with 1 cup of stemmed (see box, page 96) and finely chopped Swiss chard (any variety), packed.
- Replace the carrots with 1 cup of peeled and diced parsnips or potatoes.
- Omit the kale and zucchini. After the carrots and rice have cooked for 18 minutes, add 1 cup of chopped baby spinach, packed, and 1 cup of diced red bell pepper. Cover and cook until the vegetables and rice are tender, 3 to 5 minutes. Proceed as directed.

Creamy Lentil and Coconut Soup

Light coconut milk adds rich creaminess to this flavor-packed soup, mellowing the acidity of the tomatoes and blending beautifully with the earthy lentils. The warming spices make this soup ideal for chilly or wet weather.

1 can (15 ounces) **no-salt-added lentils, rinsed well and drained**

1 can (14 to 15 ounces) **no-salt-added diced tomatoes, with juice**

1 can (13.5 ounces; 1⅔ cups) **light coconut milk**

½ cup water

1 tablespoon garlic-infused olive oil

2 teaspoons ground cumin

2 teaspoons peeled and grated fresh ginger

1 teaspoon dried oregano

1 teaspoon paprika

½ teaspoon crushed red pepper flakes

¼ teaspoon ground cinnamon

¼ teaspoon ground turmeric

Sea salt

Freshly ground black pepper

Fresh cilantro leaves, for garnish

MAKES 4 SERVINGS

Per serving:
226 calories
8 g protein
10 g fat (4 g sat)
24 g carbs
51 mg sodium
49 mg calcium
10 g fiber

Put the lentils, tomatoes, coconut milk, water, oil, cumin, ginger, oregano, paprika, red pepper flakes, cinnamon, and turmeric in a medium soup pot (preferably nonstick) and bring to a simmer over medium-high heat. Decrease the heat to medium and cook, uncovered, stirring occasionally, until slightly thickened and the flavors have married, about 20 minutes. Adjust the heat as necessary to maintain a constant simmer. Season with salt and pepper to taste. Serve hot, garnished with fresh cilantro leaves.

Note: Analysis doesn't include sea salt or freshly ground black pepper to taste.

GINGER AND IBS

Ginger is a rhizome (a root or underground stem) that's used as a culinary seasoning as well as a natural medicinal. The phenolic compounds in ginger can aid a variety of digestive problems, including nausea, loss of appetite, dyspepsia, gas, bloating, diarrhea, constipation, gastrointestinal inflammation, and stomach pain. Although ginger can be quite peppery and hot to the taste, it calms rather than irritates the digestive system, which makes it a valuable seasoning in gut-soothing recipes.

Jarred organic ginger paste (such as The Ginger People's organic minced ginger, available in natural food stores and online) is wonderfully convenient and highly recommended. Use it in any recipe calling for peeled and grated fresh ginger.

In addition to adding ginger to foods on a regular basis, try sipping ginger tea throughout the day. It's easy to make your own. For each cup of boiling water, add 2 to 4 slices of fresh ginger. Cover and let steep for 15 minutes. Remove the ginger slices and enjoy. If desired, add a squeeze of lemon or lightly sweeten with sugar or stevia. Ginger tea is most soothing when hot or warm, but it can also be prepared in bulk and served chilled over ice.

Cream of Carrot and Parsnip Soup

MAKES 4 SERVINGS

Per serving:

275 calories

6 g protein

14 g fat (6 g sat)

34 g carbs

549 mg sodium

86 mg calcium

8 g fiber

In this recipe, carrots and parsnips are cooked with potato and then puréed into a soup that's rich and creamy, even though it contains no dairy products. The fresh ginger infuses the vegetables with spicy depth and warmth (see tip). Use any combination of carrots and parsnips that you like. The beautiful color of this soup and the eye-catching garnishes make it an elegant choice for company or a personal treat if you're dining alone.

SOUP

1½ pounds mixed carrots and parsnips, peeled and cut into 2-inch pieces

3½ cups water or Good-to-Your-Gut Vegetable Stock (page 58)

1 large potato, peeled and coarsely chopped

2 tablespoons garlic-infused olive oil

1½ tablespoons light brown sugar or unbleached cane sugar

1 tablespoon peeled and grated fresh ginger, or 1 teaspoon ground ginger

1 teaspoon dried thyme, well crushed between your fingers, or dill weed

½ teaspoon sea salt, plus more as needed

½ teaspoon freshly ground black pepper

¼ teaspoon cayenne (optional)

1 cup light coconut milk

GARNISHES (choose one, two, or all three)

8 strips Tempeh Bacon (page 49)**, whole or crumbled**

2 tablespoons chopped fresh flat-leaf parsley, lightly packed

2 tablespoons thinly sliced chives or scallion greens

Put the carrots and parsnips in a large soup pot. Add the water, potato, oil, brown sugar, ginger, thyme, salt, pepper, and optional cayenne and bring to a boil over medium-high heat. Decrease the heat to medium-low, cover, and simmer until the carrots and parsnips are very soft and the potato is tender and starting to fall apart, 50 to 60 minutes. Process with an immersion blender until smooth. Alternatively, process in batches in a high-speed blender and return to the soup pot. Stir in the coconut milk and heat through. Season with additional salt to taste. Top with the garnishes of your choice before serving.

TIP Because of the large amount of ginger used in this recipe, combined with black pepper and optional cayenne, this soup is exceedingly spicy. For a milder soup, decrease the ginger to 1 to 2 teaspoons of fresh ginger or ½ teaspoon of ground ginger, decrease the black pepper to ¼ teaspoon, and omit the cayenne.

Note: Analysis includes all three garnishes.

Facing page: Cream of Carrot and Parsnip Soup with Tempeh Bacon (page 49)

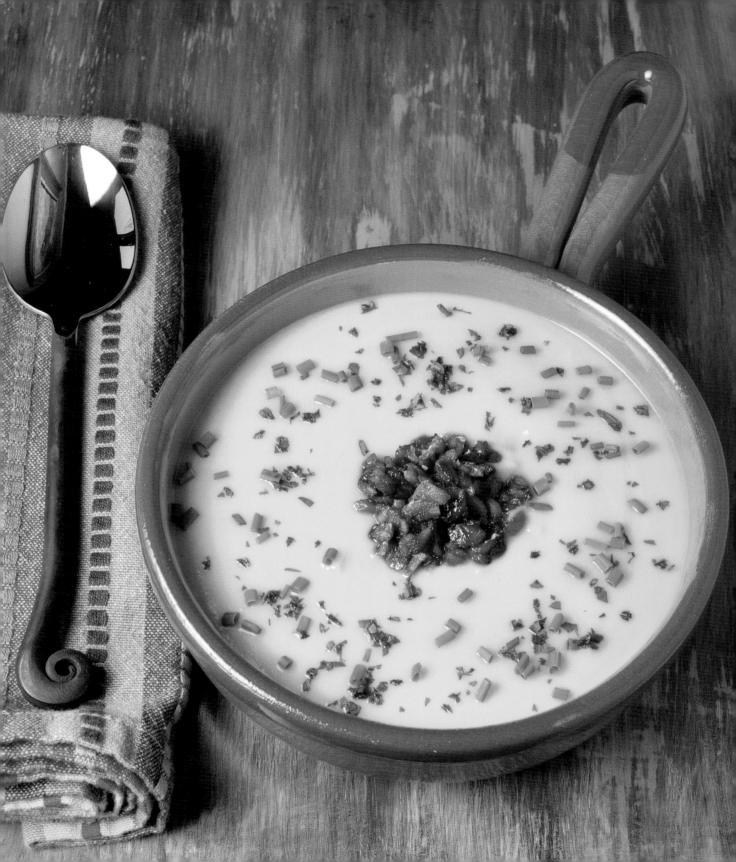

Garden Vegetable Soup

MAKES 5 SERVINGS

Per serving:

138 calories

6 g protein

1 g fat (0.1 g sat)

31 g carbs

243 mg sodium

50 mg calcium

5 g fiber

This light, brothy, fat-free soup features a colorful blend of fresh and frozen vegetables and a flavorful tomato-based stock enhanced with herbs.

3 cups water or Good-to-Your-Gut Vegetable Stock (page 58)

1 can (28 ounces) **no-salt-added crushed tomatoes, with juice**

1½ cups coarsely chopped green cabbage

1½ cups thinly sliced half-moon carrots

1½ cups peeled and cubed potatoes (½-inch cubes)

1½ cups peeled and cubed root vegetables, such as celeriac, parsnips, rutabaga, or turnips (½-inch cubes)

1 zucchini or yellow squash, cut into quarters lengthwise and sliced, or 2 patty pan squash, diced

1 cup frozen cut green beans

1½ tablespoons All-Purpose Herb Blend (page 55) **or other low-FODMAP seasoning blend**

1½ teaspoons sweet or smoked paprika

1 bay leaf

Sea salt

Freshly ground black pepper

Put the water, tomatoes, cabbage, carrots, potatoes, root vegetables, zucchini, green beans, herb blend, paprika, and bay leaf in a large soup pot and bring to a boil over high heat. Decrease the heat to medium-low, cover, and cook, stirring occasionally, until the vegetables are very tender, 30 to 40 minutes. Season with salt and pepper to taste. Remove the bay leaf before serving.

Minestrone Add 1¼ cups of canned chickpeas, rinsed well and drained, and ⅔ cup of gluten-free macaroni or other small pasta after the soup has cooked for 20 minutes.

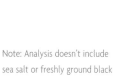

Note: Analysis doesn't include sea salt or freshly ground black pepper to taste.

Facing page: Minestrone

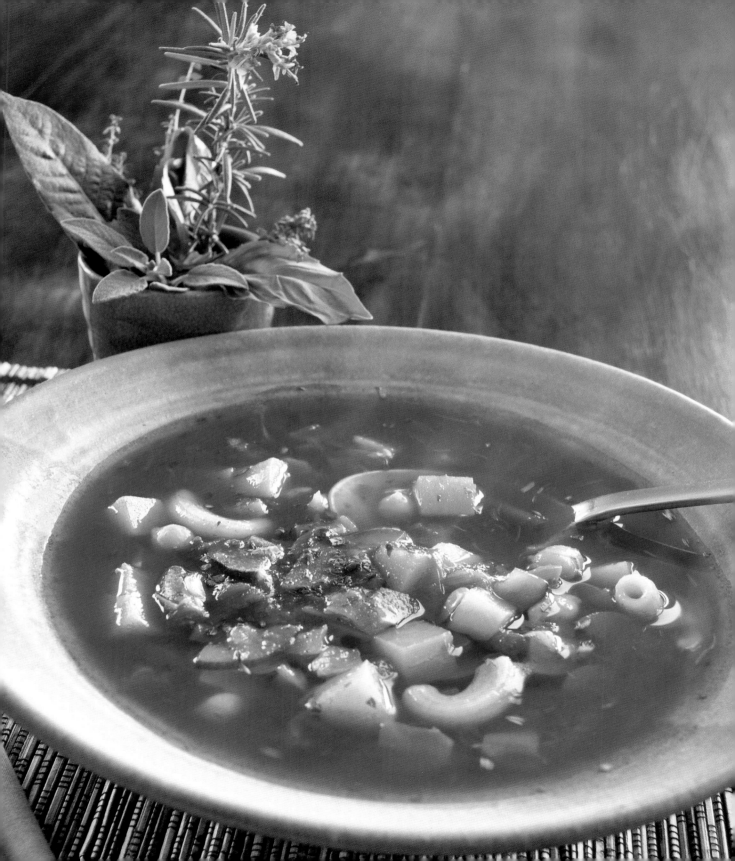

Triple-Play Veggie Sandwich

MAKES 1 SANDWICH

Per serving:

446 calories

21 g protein

21 g fat (2 g sat)

45 g carbs

674 mg sodium

235 mg calcium

5 g fiber

This three-vegetable sandwich is surprisingly hearty and adaptable. Use your favorite veggies or whatever you have on hand or need to use up. Pack it in your lunchbox or take it on a picnic. For a lighter version, use two large romaine lettuce leaves instead of the bread.

BREAD AND SPREAD

2 slices 100% sourdough spelt or wheat bread or gluten-free vegan bread

1 tablespoon vegan mayonnaise

2 teaspoons yellow mustard

Freshly ground black pepper (optional)

OPTIONAL BASE (choose one, if desired)

2 ounces Barbecued Tempeh Short Ribs (page 88)

3 ounces Barbecued Tofu Short Ribs (page 88)

3 ounces Chickenless Chicken (page 52)

2 ounces Ginger-Glazed Tempeh Filets (page 87)

3 ounces Lemon-Pepper Tofu (page 50)

½ cup thinly sliced seitan

2 ounces Tempeh Bacon (page 49)

3 ounces Tofu Bacon Strips or Slabs (page 49)

1 slice (20 grams) **low-FODMAP commercial vegan cheese**

RED VEGGIES (choose one)

4 thinly sliced rings red bell pepper

1 large red radish, thinly sliced

3 thin slices tomato

OTHER VEGGIES (choose one)

2 tablespoons shredded carrot

½ mini English cucumber, thinly sliced

3 green or black olives, thinly sliced

6 slices Zucchini in a Pickle (page 59)

¼ zucchini, very thinly sliced

LEAFY GREENS (choose one)

¼ cup alfalfa sprouts

¼ cup baby arugula, packed

¼ cup bean sprouts

¼ cup baby kale, packed

¼ cup cold cooked kale, squeezed very dry

¼ cup torn or shredded romaine lettuce, or 1 leaf romaine lettuce

¼ cup mesclun, packed

¼ cup baby spinach, packed

Put the mayonnaise and mustard in a small bowl or measuring cup and stir to combine. Spread one side of each bread slice evenly with the mayonnaise mixture. Sprinkle with pepper if desired. Over the spread on one bread slice put a layer of the optional base, followed by a layer of one red veggie option, then a layer of one other veggie option, and finally a layer of one leafy green option. Cover with the other bread slice, spread-side in. Slice on the diagonal and serve immediately.

Variation Replace the spread with 2 tablespoons of Dilled Lemon-Caper Sauce (page 82), Fresh Basil Pesto (page 112) or any of the pesto variations, Lemon-Tahini Spread (page 115), Remoulade Sauce (page 84), Sriracha Mayo (page 56), or Sriracha-Mustard Mayo (page 56).

Note: Analysis includes Lemon-Pepper Tofu (page 50), radishes, cucumber, and arugula.

Two-Way Tempeh Salad

Everyone clamors for more of this chunky salad, loaded with meaty tempeh in a creamy, herbaceous dressing. It's great on low-FODMAP crackers or in sandwiches made with 100% sourdough spelt or wheat bread or gluten-free vegan bread. For an attractive luncheon, scoop the salad onto lettuce-lined plates, garnish it with a little paprika, and surround it with fresh tomato wedges and/or pickled vegetables (see page 59). The two-way twist comes with the seasoning options: cilantro or parsley and curry powder or poultry seasoning. Take your pick and make it your way!

MAKES 4 SERVINGS

Per serving:

305 calories

11 g protein

24 g fat (2 g sat)

8 g carbs

244 mg sodium

93 mg calcium

1 g fiber

8 ounces tempeh, cut crosswise into four equal pieces

1 cup shredded carrots

½ cup vegan mayonnaise

¼ cup thinly sliced scallion greens, or 4 teaspoons dried chives

¼ cup minced fresh cilantro or flat-leaf parsley, lightly packed

1 tablespoon spicy brown or Dijon mustard, plus more as needed

1 teaspoon freshly squeezed lemon juice, plus more as needed

½ teaspoon curry powder or poultry seasoning

Sea salt

Freshly ground black pepper

Put the tempeh in a medium saucepan. Cover with water and bring to a gentle simmer over medium-high heat. Decrease the heat to medium-low and simmer gently for 10 minutes. Drain well and pat dry. Let cool, then cut into ¼-inch cubes.

Transfer the tempeh to a medium bowl and add the carrots, mayonnaise, scallion greens, cilantro, mustard, lemon juice, and curry powder. Stir gently until well combined. Add more mustard and/or lemon juice to taste if desired. Season with salt and pepper to taste. Serve at room temperature or thoroughly chilled.

Variation Add Pickle Relish (page 59) to taste.

Note: Analysis doesn't include sea salt or freshly ground black pepper to taste.

Warm Thai Noodle Salad

Warm noodle salad loaded with crunchy veggies and tossed with a spicy dressing is irresistible. It makes a sublime addition to a buffet or party meal as a first course or main dish.

MAKES 4 SERVINGS

Per serving:

662 calories

17 g protein

30 g fat (5 g sat)

89 g carbs

195 mg sodium

60 mg calcium

7 g fiber

DRESSING AND NOODLES

½ cup no-salt-added creamy or crunchy peanut butter

1 tablespoon balsamic vinegar

1 tablespoon rice vinegar or additional balsamic vinegar

1 tablespoon reduced-sodium tamari

1 tablespoon toasted sesame oil

1 tablespoon garlic-infused olive oil

1 tablespoon freshly squeezed lemon or lime juice

2 teaspoons peeled and grated fresh ginger, or ½ teaspoon ground ginger

1 teaspoon pure maple syrup

Water, as needed

Thai Red Curry Paste (page 54), **Mild Hot Sauce** (page 54), **Good-to-Your-Gut Sriracha Sauce** (page 56), **or Tabasco**

Sea salt

12 ounces gluten-free spaghetti

VEGETABLE ADDITIONS (choose four)

1 cup bean sprouts

½ cup matchstick-sliced bell peppers (any color)

½ cup finely shredded red or green cabbage

½ cup shredded carrots

½ cup matchstick-sliced English cucumber

½ cup thinly sliced, half-moon sliced, or matchstick-sliced red radishes

½ cup thinly sliced, matchstick-sliced, or diced water chestnuts

TOPPINGS (choose one, two, or all three)

½ cup chopped fresh cilantro or flat-leaf parsley, lightly packed

½ cup sliced scallion greens or chives

¼ cup Toasted Pumpkin or Sunflower Seeds (page 53), **Seasoned Pumpkin or Sunflower Seeds** (page 53), **or chopped or crushed unsalted roasted peanuts**

To make the dressing, put the peanut butter, balsamic vinegar, rice vinegar, tamari, sesame oil, garlic-infused oil, lemon juice, ginger, and maple syrup in a large bowl. Stir vigorously until smooth and well combined. Gradually whisk in enough water (about ¾ cup) to make a fairly thick but pourable sauce, beating vigorously after each addition until completely smooth. Season with curry paste and salt to taste.

To make the noodles, cook the spaghetti in boiling water according to the package directions and drain well. Add to the bowl with the sauce along with the vegetable additions of your choice and toss until the noodles are coated and the vegetables are evenly distributed. Taste and add more salt and curry paste if desired. Garnish with cilantro and/or scallion greens and sprinkle the seeds or peanuts over the top if using.

Note: Analysis includes bean sprouts, bell peppers, cabbage, carrots, cilantro, scallions, and peanuts, but doesn't include Thai Red Curry Paste or sea salt to taste.

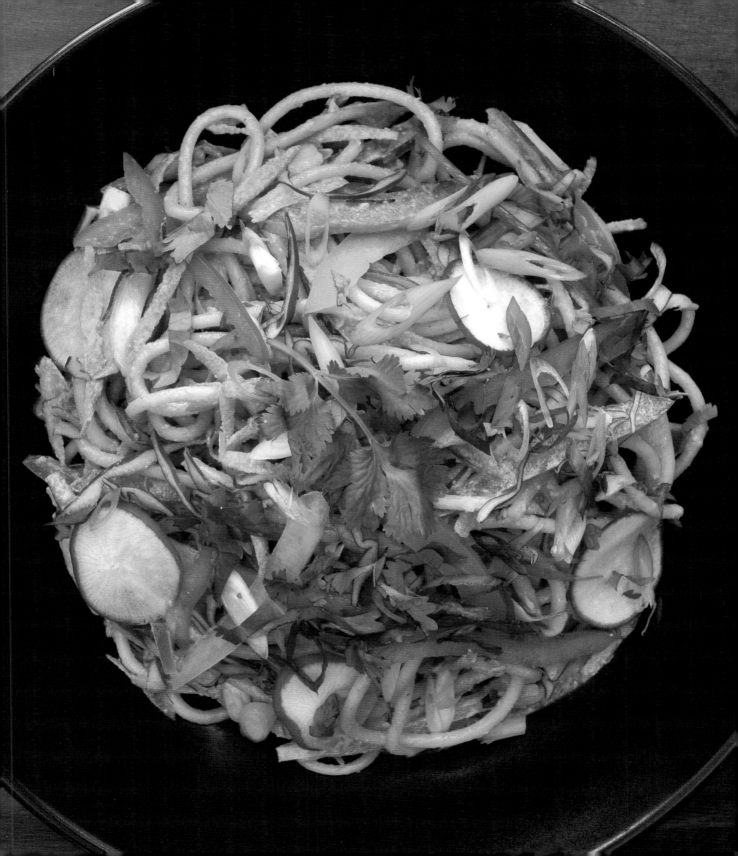

Lentil Salad with Chard and Tomatoes

MAKES 4 SERVINGS

Per serving:

288 calories

18 g protein

13 g fat (8 g sat)

26 g carbs

355 mg sodium

141 mg calcium

12 g fiber

Nutrient-dense leafy greens and protein-rich lentils make a sublime combination. Infused with flavor from the fresh ingredients and bright seasonings, then topped with tofu feta, this salad will delight even the most persnickety palate or temperamental tummy.

1 tablespoon extra-virgin olive oil

3 cups stemmed (see box, page 96) **and coarsely chopped Swiss chard** (any variety), **firmly packed**

1 can (15 ounces) **no-salt-added lentils, rinsed well and drained**

2 large tomatoes, seeded and coarsely chopped

¼ cup sliced scallion greens

2 tablespoons freshly squeezed lemon juice

1 tablespoon garlic-infused olive oil

½ teaspoon dried oregano

Sea salt

Freshly ground black pepper

1 cup coarsely crumbled Greek Tofu Feta (page 48)

Put the extra-virgin olive oil in a large skillet and heat over medium-high heat. When hot, add the chard, stir to coat with the oil, and cook, stirring almost constantly, just until wilted, 2 to 3 minutes. Transfer to a large bowl. Add the lentils, tomatoes, scallion greens, lemon juice, garlic-infused oil, and oregano and toss gently until well combined. Season with salt and pepper to taste and toss again gently. Serve immediately or thoroughly chilled. Top with the feta just before serving.

Lentil Salad with Spinach and Tomatoes Replace the Swiss chard with 3 cups of stemmed and coarsely chopped baby spinach, firmly packed.

Note: Analysis doesn't include sea salt or freshly ground black pepper to taste.

Spinach, Tomato, and Pesto Sandwich

MAKES 1 SANDWICH

Per sandwich:

401 calories

12 g protein

15 g fat (2 g sat)

54 g carbs

627 mg sodium

77 mg calcium

5 g fiber

This sandwich is a gourmet treat. You won't feel your low-FODMAP vegan diet is lacking in anything once you take a bite of this unbeatable combination. If you have access to fresh summer basil for the pesto and a tomato straight off the vine, all the better.

2 slices 100% sourdough spelt or wheat bread or gluten-free vegan bread

2 tablespoons Fresh Basil Pesto, Arugula-Spinach Pesto, Cilantro Pesto, or Kale Pesto (page 112)

1 tomato, thickly sliced

¼ cup baby spinach, firmly packed

¼ cup alfalfa sprouts (optional)

Spread one side of each bread slice evenly with the pesto. Over the spread on one bread slice put a layer of the tomato, followed by a layer of the spinach, and finally a layer of the optional sprouts. Cover with the other bread slice, spread-side in. Slice on the diagonal and serve immediately.

Spinach, Tomato, and Hummus Sandwich Replace the pesto with 2 tablespoons of Lentil Hummus, Lentil-Chickpea Hummus, or Zucchini Hummus (page 61).

Spinach, Tomato, and Pâté Sandwich Replace the pesto with 2 tablespoons of Curried Walnut Pâté, Green Bean and Walnut Pâté, Lentil and Walnut Pâté, Pecan Pâté, or Walnut Pâté (page 62).

Baby Kale and Berry Salad

Baby kale is not only a nutritional powerhouse, but it's also much sweeter and more tender than mature kale, making it a fantastic salad green. When combined with berries and pine nuts, kale is elevated beyond its well-established superfood status. This salad is low in FODMAPs but loaded with taste as well as plentiful antioxidants, calcium, and vitamins A, C, and K.

6 cups baby kale, lightly packed

1 cup blueberries, raspberries, or sliced strawberries

¼ cup pine nuts, lightly toasted (see tip, page 111)

⅓ cup Poppy Seed Dressing (page 117)

MAKES 4 SERVINGS

Per serving:
217 calories
4 g protein
16 g fat (2 g sat)
15 g carbs
118 mg sodium
76 mg calcium
3 g fiber

Put the kale, blueberries, and pine nuts in a large bowl. Whisk the dressing, pour over the salad, and toss until evenly distributed. Serve immediately.

Baby Kale and Melon Salad Replace the berries with 1 cup of diced cantaloupe or honeydew melon.

Baby Kale and Pineapple Salad Replace the berries with 1 cup of diced fresh or canned pineapple packed in juice, drained.

Variation Replace the pine nuts with toasted walnuts or pecans (see page 53) or plain Toasted Pumpkin or Sunflower Seeds (page 53).

RESOURCES

References

Chang, Lin. "The Association of Irritable Bowel Syndrome and Fibromyalgia." UNC Center for Functional GI & Motility Disorders, Chapel Hill, NC, accessed May 20, 2016, goo.gl/N0j0Z5.

Drossman, Douglas A., et al. "Rome III Diagnostic Criteria for Functional Gastrointestinal Disorders." Appendix A in *Rome III: The Functional Gastrointestinal Disorders*, 3rd ed., 885–897. MacLean, VA: Degnon Associates, Inc., 2006, romecriteria.org/assets/pdf/19_RomeIII_apA_885-898.pdf.

"Irritable-Bowel Syndrome: The Latest Irritable-Bowel Syndrome Research from Prestigious Universities and Journals Throughout the World." *Medical News Today,* [October] 2015, medicalnewstoday.com/categories/ibs.

"Migraine, Tension Headaches, and Irritable Bowel Linked?" American Academy of Neurology press release, February 23, 2016, https://goo.gl/fBjMya.

Monash University. Low FODMAP Diet smartphone app. Accessed May 20, 2016, goo.gl/0SmhYb.

Monash University. *Low FODMAP Diet for Irritable Bowel Syndrome* (blog), fodmapmonash.blogspot.com.

Shepherd, Sue, and Peter Gibson. *The Complete Low-Fodmap Diet.* New York: The Experiment, 2013.

Spiller, R., et al. "Guidelines on the Irritable Bowel Syndrome: Mechanisms and Practical Management." *Gut* 56 (2007): 1770–1798, bsg.org.uk/pdf_word_docs/ibs.pdf.

Wild, David. "Probiotic Effective for IBS and Eradicates SIBO." *Gastroenterology & Endoscopy News*, March 21, 2016, http://goo.gl/2s2Tnk.

Resources

ibsvegan.com (information about being vegan with IBS)

grassrootsvegan.com (Q&As about vegan living)

Vegan Supplements

MAGNESIUM CITRATE

NOW Foods (veggie caps)

Solgar (tablets)

MAGNESIUM GLYCINATE

Solaray (veggie caps)

Solgar (tablets)

MAGNESIUM MALATE

Source Naturals (tablets)

PSYLLIUM HUSKS

NOW Foods (powder or whole husks)

Yerba Prima (veggie caps, powder, or whole husks)

Suppliers

Anthony's Goods

organic peanut flour

goo.gl/nE3Mm4

Bob's Red Mill

a wide variety of low-FODMAP pantry staples

bobsredmill.com

Crazy Richard's Pure PB

non-GMO, fat-reduced, unsweetened peanut flour

crazyrichards.com

Just Great Stuff

organic sweetened plain and chocolate powdered peanut butter

goo.gl/eNtJzC

Olive & Marlowe

pure and flavored olive oils and vinegars

oliveandmarlowe.com

Penzey's

gluten-free spices and herbs

penzeys.com

Savory Spice Shop

gluten-free asafetida and other herbs and spices

savoryspiceshop.com

Scanpan

PFOA-free nonstick cookware

surlatable.com

williams-sonoma.com
(the Williams-Sonoma professional nonstick cookware is also PFOA-free and manufactured by Scanpan)

The Olive Tap

pure and flavored olive oils and vinegars

theolivetap.com

TofuXpress

tofu press

tofuxpress.com

Truth in Olive Oil

a list of stores in North America that sell pure and flavored olive oils

http://goo.gl/tBx0S1

INDEX

Recipe titles appear in *italics*.

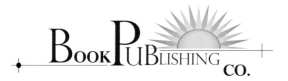

BookPublishing Co.

books that educate, inspire, and empower

To find your favorite books on plant-based cooking and nutrition,
living foods lifestyle, and healthy living,
visit BookPubCo.com

Books by Jo Stepaniak, MSEd

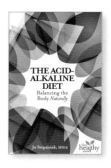

The Acid-Alkaline Diet
Jo Stepaniak, MSEd
978-1-57067-332-0 • $5.95

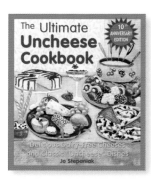

**The Ultimate
Uncheese Cookbook**
Jo Stepaniak, MSEd
978-1-57067-151-7 • $19.95

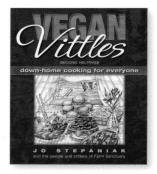

Vegan Vittles
Jo Stepaniak, MSEd
978-1-57067-200-2 • $19.95

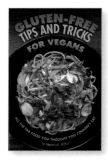

**Gluten-Free Tips
and Tricks for Vegans**
Jo Stepaniak, MSEd
978-1-57067-331-3 • $12.95

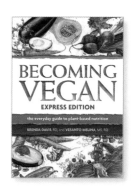

**Becoming Vegan:
Express Edition**
*Brenda Davis, RD
Vesanto Melina, MS, RD*
978-1-57067-295-8 • $19.95

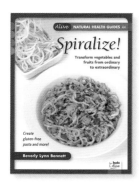

Spiralize!
Beverly Lynn Bennett
978-1-55312-052-0 • $11.95

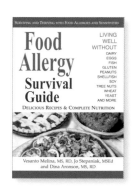

Food Allergy Survival Guide
*Vesanto Melina, MS, RD
Jo Stepaniak, MSEd
Dina Aronson, MS, RD*
978-1-57067-163-0 • $19.95

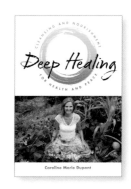

Deep Healing
Caroline Marie Dupont
978-0-92047-085-5 • $12.95

Purchase these titles from your favorite book source or buy them directly from:
Book Publishing Company • PO Box 99 • Summertown, TN 38483 • 1-888-260-8458
Free shipping and handling on all orders.